Grant Allen

AF808669

Physiological Æsthetics

Elibron Classics
www.elibron.com

Elibron Classics series.

ISBN 1-4021-7013-0 (paperback)
ISBN 1-4021-3171-2 (hardcover)

This Elibron Classics Replica Edition is an unabridged facsimile of the edition published in 1877 by Henry S. King & Co., London.

PHYSIOLOGICAL ÆSTHETICS.

PHYSIOLOGICAL ÆSTHETICS.

BY

GRANT ALLEN, B.A.

HENRY S. KING & CO., LONDON.

1877.

LONDON:
BRADBURY, AGNEW, & CO., PRINTERS, WHITEFRIARS.

TO

THE GREATEST OF LIVING PHILOSOPHERS,

HERBERT SPENCER,

I DEDICATE (BY PERMISSION)

THIS SLIGHT ATTEMPT TO EXTEND IN A SINGLE DIRECTION

THE GENERAL PRINCIPLES WHICH HE HAS LAID DOWN.

PREFACE.

"WHY we receive pleasure from some forms and colours and not from others," says Professor Ruskin, "is no more to be asked or answered than why we like sugar and dislike wormwood." The questions thus summarily dismissed by our great living authority on Æsthetics are exactly the ones which this little book asks, and, I hope, answers.

Nor is it only thinkers of Professor Ruskin's school who find a difficulty in these fundamental problems. "No doubt the perceptive powers of man and the lower animals," says Mr. Darwin, "are so constituted that brilliant colours and certain forms, as well as harmonious and rhythmical sounds, give pleasure and are called beautiful: but why this should be so we know no more than why certain bodily sensations are agreeable and others disagreeable." I have endeavoured to meet the difficulty which our great teacher thus suggests by a line of argument analogous to his own. I have attempted first to show the general relation of pleasure and pain to our organism and its circumstances; after which I have tried to prove that our existing likes and dislikes in æsthetic matters are the necessary result of natural selection.

I have had some doubt as to the proper title for my essay, which might with equal propriety be called either *physiological* or *psychological.* It is, in fact, a link of that connecting department which Mr. Herbert Spencer has well named Æstho-Physiology. Its object is to exhibit the Æsthetic Feelings as constant subjective counterparts of certain definite nervous states. But I have been influenced in the choice of that name which now appears upon the title-page by the fact that it will most clearly explain to ordinary readers the nature of my design. The subject of Æsthetics has so long been given over to transcendental rhetoric and vague poetical declamation, that the name alone upon a cover is sufficient to deter most scientific readers. I have therefore qualified it by an epithet which at once exhibits the positive point of view from which the present volume is written.

I may add, that I am not myself an excessive devotee of fine art in any form. But, on the whole, I count this as gain in attempting the psychological analysis of Æsthetics: because, as Helmholtz well observes, the worshipper of art is liable to bring with him into the consideration of its simplest elements those enthusiastic feelings which are aroused in him by its highest developments. Moreover, such a person will probably regard with contempt every species of æsthetic emotion except those most elevated ones which are capable of gratifying his own fastidious and educated taste. I have been careful, on the contrary, to seek first for an explanation of such simple pleasures in bright colour, sweet sound, or rude pictorial imitation, as delight the child and the savage; proceeding from these elementary principles to the more and more complex gratifications of natural scenery, music, painting, and poetry.

As one of my chief objects has been to economize space, I have satisfied myself in every case with the briefest and, so to speak, most diagrammatic account of physical and physiological facts. I trust this excuse will be accepted for certain simplifications of involved processes, most of which have been duly noticed in a foot-note.

My acknowledgments are due in the first and greatest degree to Mr. Herbert Spencer, and more especially to his "Principles of Psychology" and his "Essays." After these, I owe much to Professor Bain's great works on "The Senses and the Intellect," and "The Emotions and the Will." As regards the objective side of my subject, I have derived much assistance from Hermann's "Physiology." In treating of the pleasures of Hearing, I have borrowed largely from Helmholtz's "Lehre von den Tonempfindungen," translated by Mr. Ellis; and for those of Sight from the same author's "Handbuch der Physiologischen Optik," of which an English translation is still a desideratum. I have also made some use of Professor Bernstein's excellent little treatise on "The Five Senses of Man," and of Kölliker's "Manual of Human Histology."

Personally, my thanks are due to Mr. G. Coates of Baliol College, Junior Demonstrator of Physiology, and to Mr. W. W. Fisher, Aldrichian Demonstrator of Chemistry, for kind revision of my manuscript in all matters pertaining to their several departments; as well as to Mr. F. T. Richards, Lecturer of Trinity College, for much valuable assistance on psychological, philosophical, and literary points.

OXFORD, *May* 1st, 1877.

CONTENTS.

CHAPTER I.

INTRODUCTORY 1

CHAPTER II.

PLEASURE AND PAIN 5

CHAPTER III.

THE DIFFERENTIA OF ÆSTHETICS 30

CHAPTER IV.

THE LOWER SENSES 58

CHAPTER V.

TOUCH 89

CHAPTER VI.

HEARING 97

CHAPTER VII.

SIGHT 134

CHAPTER VIII.

THE INTERVENTION OF THE INTELLECT 186

CHAPTER IX.

THE IDEAL 194

CHAPTER X.

THE IMITATIVE ARTS 217

CHAPTER XI.

POETRY 243

PHYSIOLOGICAL ÆSTHETICS.

CHAPTER I.

INTRODUCTORY.

The object of the present work is to elucidate physiologically the nature of our Æsthetic Feelings. These feelings are, like all others, psychical phenomena, and our exposition must consequently take for granted in the reader a fair amount of previous knowledge in mental science generally.

The human mind falls naturally into two great divisions, the Intellect and the Emotions. The former is mainly concerned with agreement and difference, the latter with pleasure and pain. The Æsthetic Feelings belong to the emotional in contradistinction to the intellectual part of our being: that is to say, they are phenomena of pleasure and pain, not of mere neutral discrimination. Hence our first task must be to examine the nature of these fundamental emotional elements, and then to show in what manner the Æsthetic Feelings may be treated as special cases referable to their general laws. Accordingly, we will begin with an enquiry into the physical states which are the objective concomitants of pleasures and pains generally; we will then determine in what manner the special class of pleasures and pains known as æsthetic differ from the remainder of their genus; and we will finally endeavour to show that the physical states which accompany each such Æsthetic Feeling are the same in kind as those which characterize all other pleasures or pains, as the case may be, whose bodily nature is more readily recognisable.

In other words, my object is to exhibit the purely physical origin of the sense of beauty, and its relativity to our nervous organisation. Modern scientific Psychology, based upon an accurate Physiology, has roughly demonstrated that all mental phenomena are the subjective sides of what are objectively cognised as nervous functions; and that they are in consequence as rigorously limited by natural laws as the physical processes whose correlatives they are. But while this truth has been abundantly illustrated with regard to those psychical functions (such as sensations and voluntary motions) which are ordinarily regarded as of purely bodily origin, it has not been carried out into full detail in the case of the intellectual faculties and the higher emotions, which, until the rise of Physiological Psychology, were usually considered as purely and exclusively mental. I wish, therefore, to examine the Æsthetic Feelings as an intermediate link between the bodily senses and the higher emotions; and, by affiliating them upon a physiological law of pleasure and pain, to pave the way for a similar detailed treatment of the intellect and the affections. My work is thus the fuller development in a single direction of that which has been inaugurated for the whole field of Psychology by Mr. Herbert Spencer, Professor Bain, Dr. Maudsley, and other leaders in the science of mind.

The formal definition of the Æsthetic Feelings must obviously be posponed till we have previously considered the higher genus of which they form a subordinate species; for before we examine the question of pleasure and pain in general, we cannot rightly mark off the æsthetic class from the other feelings comprised under those general headings. Accordingly, the question must be deferred till the chapter on the Differentia of Æsthetics. But it will be convenient to settle provisionally in an empirical way what are the sort of phenomena with which we are ultimately to deal, and later on to substitute for this rough conception a reasoned formula. By the Æsthetic pleasures and pains we mean those which result from the contemplation of the beautiful or the ugly, in art or nature, alike in the actuality and in the idea. Of course the words *beautiful* and *ugly* are themselves mere symbols of the Æsthetic Feelings and in no way help us to form an analytic conclusion; but they are convenient for immediate use, because they convey a definite and familiar meaning, the psychological import of which must be hereafter exposed. As simple instances of the beautiful in nature, we may mention gems, flowers, birds, butterflies, and human beings, or aggregates such as the mountains, woods, streams, and valleys which compose natural scenery. In art, we may mention architecture, painting, sculpture, and music. Both these classes agree in so far as they are all beautiful in the actuality: poetry and imaginative literature supply us with the same in the ideal. So that, speaking popularly, the subject-matter of our investigation will be the feelings aroused in man by the beautiful in nature, and in the arts of architecture, painting, sculpture, music, and poetry: special attention being paid throughout to the component factors of the last. This provisional enumeration must stand for the present in place of a rational definition.

CHAPTER II.

PLEASURE AND PAIN.

§ 1. *Method of Investigation.*

The Æsthetic Feelings being a special class of Pleasures and Pains, we begin, as proposed, by investigating the nature of Pleasures and Pains generally; and we shall afterwards endeavour to show wherein those which are known as æsthetic differ from the remainder of their respective genera.

The usual method pursued in abstract subjects is, first, to state the main conclusions at which the author has arrived, and then to detail the particular instances upon which they are based. Occasionally, however, it is expedient to reverse this process, so as first to examine the phenomena under investigation, and then to draw from them the generalizations which they suggest. In approaching the difficult question of the nature of Pleasure and Pain, the latter course seems to me the most desirable, in order that the subject may be more naturally and gradually unfolded: and I shall consequently make no apology for plunging at once *in medias res* and asking the reader to follow me for a time in the dark, while I endeavour to trace out the laws of the connexion between these two antithetical modes of consciousness and the bodily states whose concomitants they are.

I do not propose to consider in the present chapter the Pleasures and Pains of the Intellect or the higher Emotions. These, as being specially-involved cases of the general laws, will receive special attention in later portions of this work. Nor shall I attempt directly to elucidate those of the Æsthetic Feelings themselves, as they will form the subject-matter of the remaining chapters of our treatise. At present I shall only deal with such Pleasures and Pains as are commonly referred to a purely bodily origin, those namely of the five senses and of the general organic and muscular sensibility; in order that from these most conspicuous examples we may infer the laws of Pleasures and Pains generally. And I shall begin with Pain, because its manifestations are more obvious and noticeable than those of the opposite feeling.

§ 2. *Pain.*

If we take a rapid survey of the principal varieties of physical Pain, the first point which strikes us is that the greater part of them, and especially the most intense, are the concomitants of a violent dismemberment in some one of the tissues. Of all Pains with which we are acquainted, the strongest are those which accompany the severance of an actual sensible portion of the body, as in the amputation of a limb, the excision of an ulcer, or the removal of a scalp. The disruption from the body of a much smaller member is also extremely painful, as, for example, the loss of a nail or the drawing of a tooth. To pinch off a small piece of skin (below the epidermis) or to pull out a hair occasions a considerable smart. In short, to tear or cut away from the body any one of its constituent tissues is one most conspicuous cause of Pain.

Again, merely to sever the tissues without actual dismemberment is also painful. Take as instances wounds, cuts, pricks, and scratches. To pare or break the nails below the quick, to pull open a sore, to have the face or lips chapped, are other similar cases. Disruption of tissue is therefore a second and closely-allied cause of Pain.

Disintegration of any part of the body owing to causes not so directly mechanical is accompanied by the same subjective states: as in burning off a finger, having the feet frozen so that the joints drop off, destroying the skin and muscles with a corrosive acid, and so forth.

Like mental manifestations occur when the tissues are bruised, crushed, or broken. Of this we have everyday experience in blows, falls, kicks, and rubs. Here we can easily see that there is still disintegration, though of smaller tissues. This is proved by the concentration of blood in the area of disruption which causes the flesh to appear "black and blue," and shows that the delicate epithelium of the capillaries has been broken and an extravasation has taken place; by the weal, raised after a smart tap from a whip; and by the blisters which follow friction, and testify to the separation of the skin from the subjacent tissues by allowing an effusion to collect in the interstice.

All these cases are produced by the interference of external bodies with the organism. But there are other cases where, owing to internal causes, portions of the body waste away in eating sores, such as abscesses, cancer, ulcers, whitlows, &c. All these are also accompanied by Pain. And, finally, there are a few cases where internal membranes give way under excessive pressure, and cause extremely painful sensations.

Now a consideration of all these instances might lead us to suspect that Pain is intimately connected with the destruction of bodily tissues; and if we continue our examination, we shall see that a large number of other phenomena, which do not at first sight seem to be manifestations of the same principle, are easily brought into conformity with it. For many painful actions, which are not conspicuously disruptive in their ordinary degree, become obviously so when pushed to an extreme. Thus, the heat of a candle held close to one's hand causes Pain, although there is no apparent disintegration; yet, inasmuch as, if we continue the action sufficiently long or hold the candle sufficiently close, disruption will be set up and made manifest by the consequent blister, we may reasonably conclude that a lesser molecular disruption had from the beginning been set up. Similarly with cold: if pushed to an extreme, disintegration will become evident; and even when it is only experienced in a moderate degree, the chapping of the skin shows that separation between its particles has taken place. The unpleasant feelings derived from tight boots, blisters on the hands from rowing, hard beds or seats, rough bodies rubbed over the skin, are all explicable in a similar manner. They culminate in corns, bunions, bed sores, and lacerations. The Pains of many diseases allow of a like explanation. Intestinal Pain is often due to the distention of the membranes by solid or gaseous matter, which must obviously result in slight ruptures or strains upon their surfaces. The passage of renal calculi, gall stones, or clotted catamenial discharges is sometimes perfectly excruciating. Ulcerated sore-throat and many other internal complaints are obviously disintegrative in their nature. Inflammatory diseases, such as gout, imply a straining of the tissues in the inflamed parts. Irritant gases, when inhaled, destroy the pulmonary tissues. Toothache is produced either by the actual exposure and wasting away of a nerve, or by virulent matter arising from decomposition of the teeth being carried to the nerve and setting up destructive chemical action. In short, a great number of Pains may be explained by very slight dismemberments of minor portions of the body.

In other cases the evidence only shows a tendency to disruption rather than its actual presence. Whenever a mass of connective tissue is exposed to a violent strain, the nerves which it contains are pinched or twisted and arouse an intensely painful sensation. Sprains, cramps, and spasms, are all due to disruptive pulls upon a muscle or tendon. Twitching the hair, jerking a limb, pinching the flesh, yield kindred feelings of less intensity. Here also we may perhaps suppose that there is actual separation of minute tissues; for if we continue pulling the hair, we pull it out; if we go on jerking the limb, we dislocate it; and if we pinch hard enough, we leave a black and blue mark. However this may be, we may for safety's sake sum up our conclusion as follows: the greater number of Pains are the subjective concomitants of an actual disruption or disruptive tendency in some one of the bodily tissues.

Here it may be objected that this principle does not account for the Pain which succeeds a wound or laceration, even after the actual dismemberment has taken place. It would seem that as soon as the destructive action ceases, the Pain should also cease. I believe that such is really the case. The Pain of a wound probably arises from oxidation and its subsequent effects, or from hard substances rubbing against the exposed nerves. It is now generally believed that decomposition results from the action of small floating germs, known as *vibrios*, and that if these can be excluded, putrefaction will not set in. If we dress a wound at once, and do not move the limb or bring it into contact with external bodies, we suffer hardly any Pain, except the weakness from excessive nerve-action and loss of blood, of which more hereafter.* When, on the contrary, we expose it to the air, inflammation sets in, and results in openly disintegrative action. If, after removing a cantharides blister, we apply a cloth covered with cold-cream, the Pain is immediately allayed. If we allow the rough edges of our clothing to rub against the raw surface, it becomes extremely painful. Burns and scalds scarcely give any trouble if the part affected is covered, and the air excluded immediately.

* See Mr. James Hinton's essays "On Rest and Pain."

If, on the contrary, in addition to exposing a wound or burn, we also rub upon it bodies which are known to act chemically upon the tissues, such as salt or pepper, the painfulness is greatly increased. Probably the oxygen of the air acts in the same manner, only to a less extent. So we may conclude as a rule that the continued painfulness of wounds is due to continued destruction of tissue taking place unperceived.

It may be further objected that many destructive actions are not accompanied by painful feelings. Cutting or burning the hair; running a pin through the outer skin of the fingers; paring, scraping, or corroding with acids the nails, horns, or hoofs, yield no emotional counterparts whatsoever. To this, of course, the simple morphological answer can be given that the epidermis, with its various modifications, is not supplied with nerves, and as all consciousness is the correlative of nervous changes, these parts add nothing directly to its sum. For the mass of animals who must constantly come into contact with slightly destructive agencies in the environment, it is obviously desirable that the body should be protected by such a non-sensitive sheath. But the moment we attempt to remove entirely these protective membranes, to tear off the nails, to flay alive, to pull out the hair, to draw a tooth, we arrive at tissues copiously supplied with nerves, and violent Pain is set up, inducing of course a cessation from the action if it be voluntary, or resistance to it if it be the work of another organism. But it may be further said that in some internal maladies, such as phthisis and various diseases of the heart and liver, considerable disintegration often takes place before the patient experiences painful sensations. Here we have to deal with viscera mainly supplied with nerves from the sympathetic ganglia, or possessing independent systems of their own, and inasmuch as, in the vertebrata, the cerebro-spinal system is the sole seat of consciousness, it follows that Pain can only be felt in these organs when the disintegration reaches portions of them or of adjacent tissues which are supplied with cerebro-spinal fibres. The inter-communication between the two systems is, however, so intimate and intricate that internal diseases exhibit the greatest apparent capriciousness in their painful or painless character. Lastly, direct experiment has shown that if the cut end of an *efferent* nerve in unbroken connexion with the brain be irritated, no consciousness of any sort ensues. We may therefore add to our previous rough generalization the limiting clause—provided the tissue be supplied with afferent cerebro-spinal nerves in unbroken connexion with the brain.

But does this generalization include all classes of Pains, and if not, to which particular species does it apply? Professor Bain has well divided Pains into two main classes, the Massive and the Acute. The former are those which arise from affections of the whole organism, or large tracts of it, and are weak in intensity: the latter, those which arise from affections of special limited areas, and are strong in intensity. Now the above enumerated Pains, which have for their physical antecedent a disintegration of tissue, belong for the most part to the Acute class. It is to this class that the principle is mainly applicable, and we may sum it up in the following law and corollary: Acute Pains are the subjective feelings which accompany an actual disruption or disruptive tendency in a tissue supplied with afferent cerebro-spinal nerves in unbroken communication with the brain; the *degree of acuteness* of such Pains varying with the violence and completeness of the disruption, and their *amounts* varying with the size of the area affected.* The truth of the corollary will be recognised if we remember the sharpness of the smart which is produced by pulling out a hair or tearing a small piece of skin off the back of the fingers, and then contrast its volume with that which is experienced on breaking a limb or undergoing a severe surgical operation.

The Acute Pains which we have hitherto considered are those belonging to the general sensibility of the body. But can the same principle be extended to the Pains of the special senses? We must run through them briefly in detail, and see to what conclusions our observations will lead us.

Beginning with Taste, we know that those pungent and acid substances which produce irritation of the tongue are capable of disintegrating the tissues. Mustard or cayenne pepper in excess are painful; and either of them, if moistened and laid on any part of the skin, soon gives rise

* In anticipation of a minor criticism it may be well to add that the Pain is, more strictly speaking, proportionate to the number of nerves severed or strained; and that the peripheral end-organs, when injured, yield far more Pain than the nerve fibres on their course.

to destructive action, as shown by the ensuing blister. The larger and more exposed nerve-terminations of the tongue render it more rapidly sensible than other portions of the body: in other words, the destructive action is probably set up there much more instantaneously then elsewhere. Alkalies, everywhere disintegrative, specially affect the oral cavity. We have no direct evidence as to the action of bitter substances, but reasons will be adduced in a later chapter, which render it probable that they are similarly destructive to the nerve-terminations. Other unpleasant tastes will receive more extended treatment in the same place.

In Smell, the tactual nerves distributed to the entrance of the respiratory canal are affected by pungent odours (such as ammonia) in the same manner as those of the tongue by pungent tastes. If the smallness in amount of the irritant seems inconsistent with the notion of disintegration, we must remember that the special sense-organs are collections of specially-unstable nerve-matter, so placed as to be specially disturbed by small incident energies, and that this indeed constitutes their very essence as specialized organs. The case of smells proper will form the subject of a separate section later on; but there is nothing improbable in the conjecture that the disagreeable ones destructively attack the olfactory cells.

Touch yields us hardly any Pains; but the unpleasant sensation produced by a rough object in contact with the skin and chafing against it is evidently a result of slight disintegrative tendencies.

In Hearing, it is clear that very loud sounds, such as the

boom of a cannon, will cause an excessive waste of nervous tissue, accompanied by a corresponding Pain. So, too, will sounds which recur with extreme frequency, or which are continued for very long periods. Hence the disagreeable effect of crashes, bangs, monotony, or constant noise.

Sight yields us like illustrations. Brilliant lights, as those of the sun or the voltaic arc, are the exact analogues of loud sounds, and involve excessive waste of tissue. Masses of bright colour, monotony of hue, sparkling objects like snow or ice, demand prolonged and wearisome exercise. But these cases fall more naturally under the second or Massive division of Pains, among which fatigue is to be reckoned. To these, then, we next proceed.

Besides the Acute feelings which are given by dismemberments of the body, we are all familiar with another class of disagreeable sensations whose distinguishing subjective feature is lassitude or want of vigour. The principal varieties are, fatigue after muscular exertion ; mental weariness ; inanition from want of food ; faintness from anæmia, loss of blood, sleeplessness, or over-exertion ; weakness from fever or other depressing disease ; nervous debility ; and those undefinable organic feelings which result from general ill-health. This whole class is strongly marked off from the preceding one both subjectively and objectively. On the psychical side, the vivid element of Pain proper is wanting, and there is present in its stead a vaguer feeling of distress. Indeed, the class might better be described as Discomforts than as Pains, only that unfortunately we have no more comprehensive term under which to include them both. On the physical side, they result rather from a want of efficiency in the tissues than from any actual disintegration. The Acute Pains, as a class, arise from the action of surrounding destructive agencies; the Massive Pains as a class, from excessive function or insufficient nutriment. Of course, wounds and amputations cause loss of blood, and so give rise to Massive Pains; while, on the other hand, many diseases are accompanied by Acute Pains: still, in each case, the sufferer is able easily to distinguish between the two sets of feelings, and to refer them accurately to their objective counterparts.

Massive Pains are occasioned by a general state of innutrition, either in the body as a whole or in any of its component systems. The organism being perpetually disintegrated by slow degrees, as its de-energized constituents are cast off and excreted, requires to be supplied with fresh integrable energy-yielding matter from time to time: and if it is not, the unpleasant feelings of inanition and faintness occur. When muscular toil has been pushed too far, a disintegration takes place beyond the regular repairing powers of the circulating fluids, and the result is the feeling of fatigue. In a wound, besides the Acute Pain of the disruption, there is loss of blood and waste of nerve tissue, both of which conspire to produce faintness. In febrile disorders, the energy-yielding tissues are wastefully consumed, and the loss gives rise to weakness and giddiness. In the special organs, over-use is followed by fatigue, as in reading too long, looking at a bright light or a mass of white, hearing a din or roar, and so forth. In the brain, excessive thought is followed by depression. In short, Massive Discomforts occur whenever, in the whole or any part, waste of tissue largely outruns repair; and this may happen alike from rapidity of waste or from insufficiency of repairing matter.

It should also be noted that Massive Pains, when pushed to an extreme, merge into the Acute class. For example, the gnawing feelings of inanition, the burning of thirst, and the excessive stimulation of the eye or ear, all reach a pitch of painfulness which may well be considered as Acute. Neuralgia is also attributed by most modern authorities to a general state of innutrition in the nervous system or a portion of it. Indeed, the two classes are rather indefinite in their limits, being simply a convenient working distinction, not a natural division.

In order to account for the nexus between these objective states and their subjective manifestations, the human or animal organism may be conveniently regarded as a complicated and delicate machine, specially constructed for self-conservation and the production of like organisms in the future. That it should be so constructed as to correspond with the environment is a condition-precedent of its existence at all. Hence every organism, in proportion to the completeness of its adaptation, energetically resists any act which interferes with its efficiency as a working machine: and such interferences are known subjectively as Pains. Now nothing can more thoroughly militate against the efficiency of the mechanism than the loss of any one of its component parts: and we find accordingly that to deprive the body of any one of its members is painful in a degree roughly proportionate to the general value of such member to the organism as a whole. Take for example the relative painfulness of severing from the body a leg, an arm, an eye, a finger-nail, a hair, or a piece of skin. Acute Pains are those which arise from any such dismemberment of the working machine: and, the organism being self-regulating, they naturally prompt to the most energetic efforts for the cessation or suppression of the destructive action.

Again, the body being a machine, and all machines being devices for the transference of potential into kinetic energy, it is necessary that the body should from time to time be supplied with matters possessing potential energy. It is accordingly fatal to the organism that it should not be sufficiently supplied with the matters necessary for replacing the losses which it sustains in performing its functions. For when once the organism ceases entirely from the cycle of its functions, they are seldom if ever restored.* So, too, it is in a lesser degree undesirable that any part should be so rapidly disintegrated as to outrun the supply of energy-yielding matters afforded it by the blood. Hence arise Massive Pains; which, when caused by fatigue, partial or general, lead us to seek that repose which alone can give relief and restore the wasted tissues; and, when caused by the lack of integrable matter, prompt us, through the feelings which we class as *cravings* or *appetites*, to search after the needful objects of food and drink.

* I make the exception in favour of recoveries from what is dogmatically termed "suspended animation."

An illustration of an extreme sort will make this clear. If we suppose locomotive engines to have been evolved by natural selection, instead of having been consciously produced by the art of man; and if we imagine them to be in the habit of finding the coal for their own furnaces, and the water for their own boilers; if we further conceive them to supply automatically, by circulating ducts, the losses through friction in their joints, and to spread oil over their bearings; and if, lastly, we crown the picture by supposing these grotesque and complicated monsters to be endowed with consciousness similar to our own: then, upon any attempt to hack or destroy the piston or cylinder, to oxydise any portion of the fittings, or to pull asunder any of the joints, the engine would experience a feeling analogous to Acute Pain, and would make violent demonstrations of resistance; upon any deficiency of water or coal, interfering with its proper working, it would be the subject of a Massive Discomfort, in the shape of a craving, which would prompt it to seek the missing element; while, lastly, upon any considerable waste of its substance or extra friction from want of oil, it would suffer from the other variety of Massive Pain, known as fatigue, which would produce an inaction, analogous to sleep, until the automatic circulation had repaired the wasted parts and supplied the lost lubricating matter. Such self-conserving machines are all living organisms; and, unless they were so, they would necessarily cease to exist themselves, and would be unable to produce similar beings for the future.

Finally, it may be added, without entering into the

ultimate question of the connexion between physical and psychical states, that there seems a certain concinnity and fitness in the correspondence between these feelings and their objective counterparts: in other words, the consciousness of Pain or Discomfort bears somewhat the same relation to other conscious states as the physical fact which underlies it bears to other conditions of the system.

§ 3. *Pleasure.*

We may now leave Pains for the present, and pass on to the consideration of Pleasures, returning to the former subject in a general summing up, which we shall be better able to understand when we have looked at both sides of our emotional nature.

Professor Bain has formulated the connexion of emotional feelings with physical states in the following law: "States of pleasure are concomitant with an increase, and states of pain with an abatement, of some, or all, of the vital functions." Now with regard to Pains, the reader will have already seen that this law is both too vague and too general, but is otherwise correct, as far as it goes. As regards Pleasures, however, it seems open to more serious objection. In the endeavour to be antithetical it misses the real relationship between the two states. If Pleasures were the psychical concomitants of an *increase* of some of the vital functions, then our two greatest, if not our only Pleasures ought to be digestion, and repose after exertion: whereas these are really only minor and very indefinite Pleasures. Mr. Bain has sighted this difficulty, but, not appreciating its full force, has endeavoured to avoid it by a supplementary theory of "stimulation," which appears to me far more important than his main law. I believe the true principle of connexion to be this: Pleasure is the concomitant of the healthy action of any or all of the organs or members supplied with afferent cerebro-spinal nerves, to an extent not exceeding the ordinary powers of reparation possessed by the system. And just as the two laws are not exactly antithetical, so, too, the feelings themselves are not directly and absolutely opposed to one another, as will be seen in the sequel.

To begin, as before, with the most obvious manifestations, Pleasure on the whole is chiefly referable to a healthy state of the organism generally, one in which every part is enabled to perform its proper functions unimpeded, and no undue call is made upon any single organ or member. It is true that in such a state of the organism we are not conscious of any special or acute Pleasure, particularly if we are not engaged in the active exercise of our limbs, or of the alimentary and sexual organs: but we *are* conscious (in the absence of any pain-giving causes) of a subdued undercurrent of pleasurable feeling which forms the background of our emotional state. And if, in such a condition of body, we give free play to all the activities of the system, nervous and muscular,—as in taking a morning walk on a sunny day in spring, after a good night's rest, and a hearty breakfast,—we receive a massive impression of Pleasure which corresponds partially to the massive discomfort of fatigue, inanition, or anæmia. Now, in the first of these cases, the faint background of

Pleasure is apparently referable to the due and unimpeded performance of the automatic energies, such as the circulatory, respiratory, and digestive functions, which here as elsewhere add only a vague and unlocalised element to consciousness: while in the second case it is due to the voluntary activity of the muscular system, and to the stimulation of the freshly-repaired end-organs of nerves. Again, when we apply the proper stimulus to those organs whose action is most intermittent (as those connected with alimentation and reproduction), we are conscious of an acute impression of Pleasure, resulting from the strong but normal excitation of fully-nurtured nervous structures. In short, it will be seen that while Professor Bain refers Pleasure to an *increase* in the efficiency of the organism, it may better be regarded as the concomitant of a *normal amount of activity* in any portion or the whole of the organism. Or, to employ once more our metaphor of the steam-engine, we may say that Pleasure results, not from the act of coaling, watering, or oiling, but from the harmonious working of all the parts. And, as all activity implies a waste of tissue (since it is dynamically equivalent to the passage of potential into kinetic energy), Pleasure is to a certain extent concomitant with a *decrease* of vital function. The limit at which such waste of tissue ceases to be pleasurable and begins to be painful is, I believe, the point where the waste exceeds the ordinary powers of repair.

A single concrete instance will help to explain this. In the muscular sensibility we see at once that Pleasure is the resultant of activity after repose. As soon, however, as the exercise has been continued to a point beyond the repairing powers of the system, Massive Pain, known as fatigue, sets in. It is true, as Mr. J. S. Mill objected, that we only know when this point has been reached by the consciousness of fatigue itself: but that does not destroy the objective character of the fact. Viewed on its physiological side, the subject may be thus stated. Our nerves and muscles are supplied with a certain relatively-fixed amount of energy-yielding matters. After every active employment of the tissue, a certain amount of these matters, equivalent to the strength of the activity, is deprived of its energy, and is cast off into the blood as a decomposition product. The quantity of energy-yielding matters contained in each tissue is, of course, greatest after the integrative periods of ingestion, sleep or repose; and least after continued exercise of the tissue, or long intermission of ingestion or reparation. The amount of energy-yielding matters available for ordinary activities lies between these two extremes. So long as a particular organ or member is called upon to yield up only so much of its energy as can be repaired within the normal period so as to restore it to its average condition, the resulting feeling is pleasurable, or at least neutral. But if it be called upon to expend so much energy as will depress it below its average condition, massive discomfort results, and increases in proportion to the extent to which the tissues are wasted. It is the same if, after the average amount of waste, new energy-yielding matters are not integrated. A starving sheep, as Professor Huxley forcibly puts it, is in the truest sense a carnivore; for it is using up, in the performance of its physiological functions, energy derived from the permanent tissues of its own organism. To borrow a metaphor from Political Economy, we may regard every tissue as possessing a normal quantity of energy-yielding matters, as a reserve fund or fixed capital, and also another quantity as wages-fund or working capital. So long as it only employs the working capital, which from day to day and from minute to minute renews itself, without ever trenching upon the reserve-fund, all goes well, and the concern works easily. But as soon as it passes this limit and begins to draw upon its reserve or spend its fixed capital, there results the consciousness of bad working in the concern which we know as Pain or discomfort.

But it is only occasionally that the general exercise of the muscles or of the sense-organs yields us a distinct feeling of Pleasure. For the most part, our activities afford us merely a neutral consciousness of the intellectual sort, without emotional differentiation. Very seldom do they rise to the intensity of recognizable Pleasures. And this is explicable enough. Doubtless, every activity, when not excessive nor of a sort to prove destructive to the tissues, is in itself faintly pleasurable;—indeed, we generally recognise this fact in our ordinary language;—but owing to the commonness and faintness of the feeling, we habitually disregard it. There are, however, two sets of occasions upon which the feeling aroused is sufficiently vivid to be recognised as distinctly pleasurable. The first is when, in a healthy state of the whole organism, under the influence of abundant food and good rest, the general stimulation of the nerves produces a consciousness of Massive Pleasure; the second is when the special stimulation of a single organ, whose periods of activity are long intermittent, and which is at the culminating point of its nutrition, produces the consciousness of Acute Pleasure.

As the Pleasures of the special senses will form the subject-matter of our future chapters, we need not enter into them fully here. It will be sufficient to point out a few minor peculiarities. The strongest Pleasures result from the stimulation of the largest nervous organs, whose activities are most intermitted, as in the case of the alimentary and reproductive senses. These Pleasures are greatest after the longest intermissions, and are scarcely felt at all if stimulations are too frequently repeated. The weakest Pleasures are those of the most universally stimulated organs, as in the tactual and thermal senses. Intermediate between these come the Pleasures of sight and hearing, which are comparatively intermittent in their activities, and whose stimulations are pleasurable in proportion to the infrequency of their occurrence. In short, the amount of Pleasure is probably in the direct ratio of the number of nerve fibres involved, and in the inverse ratio of the natural frequency of excitation.

And here we see wherein the feeling of Pleasure fails to be exactly antithetical to the feeling of Pain, just as their objective antecedents similarly fail. Massive Pleasure can seldom or never attain the intensity of Massive Pain, because the organism can be brought down to almost any point of innutrition or exhaustion, but its efficient working cannot be raised very high above the average. Similarly, any special organ or plexus of nerves can undergo any amount of violent disruption or wasting away, giving rise to extremely Acute Pains; but organs are very seldom so highly nurtured and so long deprived of their appropriate stimulant as to give rise to very Acute Pleasure. Hence the common experience that our greatest Pleasures fall far short in intensity of our greatest Pains. It is in such a rare instance alone as that of the sexual organs, where stimulation only takes place (in normal cases) after long intervals of rest and nutrition, that Pleasure rises to the same pitch of monopolising consciousness which is so ordinary a result of excessive Pain.

§ 4. *Invariability of the Relation between Pleasures or Pains and their Objective Concomitants.*

There is one final question, of great importance, which must be settled before we leave this part of our subject. It may be asked,—If Pleasure and Pain have the objective origin here assigned to them, how comes it that some deleterious acts are pleasant and some useful ones painful? Paradoxical as it may seem, the simple answer is, they are not. There are no such cases. Every act, so long as it is pleasurable, is in so far a healthy and useful one; and conversely, so long as it is painful, a morbid and destructive one. The fallacy lies in the proleptic employment of the words "deleterious" and "useful." To put it in a simple form, the nervous system is not *prophetic*. It informs us of what is its actual state at the moment, not what the after effects of that state will be. If we take sugar of lead, we receive at first a pleasant sensation of sweetness, because the immediate effect upon the nerves of taste is that of a healthy stimulation. Later on, when the poison begins to work, we are conscious of a painful sensation of griping, because the nerves of the intestines are then being actually disintegrated by the direct or indirect action of the irritant. In the process of evolution the higher organisms have gone on establishing a consensus between the various organs of the body, so that at last, for the most part, whatever will prove deleterious to any organ proves deleterious also to the first nerves of the organism which it affects; and such a harmony between the organs, once partially established, is continued and strengthened by the survival of the fittest. Naturally, however, this can only be the case when the deleterious object is found sufficiently often in the environment to give an additional point of advantage to any species which is so adapted as to discriminate and reject it. Now, acetate of lead does not occur at all frequently in nature, and moreover it closely resembles in its action upon the nerves of taste a commonly diffused and highly nutritious substance, sugar. Consequently, our nerves of taste, which have been so developed as to be normally stimulated by sugar, are similarly stimulated by the poisonous acetate. It is only when the internal nerves are acted upon that the difference begins to be perceived: and then the Pain gives an unfailing indication of disintegrative action.

Indeed, the whole development of the special senses is a

continuous adaptation of the organism to the environment, one of whose phases necessarily consists in the establishment of a consensus between the external peripheral nerves and those of the internal organs. Just as sight is a "premonitory touch," and smell a premonitory taste, so taste itself is premonitory of the effect which the food will produce upon the digestive and assimilative systems. However, such adaptation can only be approximate, at least until that final future equilibration when the organism has in every way adapted itself to every possible modification of the environment. At any point short of that ideal goal, numerous failures of adaptation must naturally occur. Amongst mankind, the intellect has to fill up the gaps in the adaptation of the senses. For instance, the child who lights upon sugar of lead will trust only to the taste as a guide to its desirability as food; the ordinary educated man will look for a label on the phial; and the instructed chemist will recognise and avoid it by observing its peculiar properties. But in every case the nerves actually stimulated faithfully reflect their existing state at the moment of observation, by the feelings of Pleasure or Pain which they yield.

§ 5. *Recapitulation.*

And now let us briefly sum up the general conclusions at which we have arrived. The human organism is a highly complex but not absolutely perfect self-regulating machine. It differs from machines of human construction in possessing the mysterious attribute of consciousness. This consciousness is specially connected with and definitely related to a certain portion of the organism, known as the cerebro-spinal nervous system: or rather with particular members of that system. Every state of consciousness is a reflex or outcome of their physical states. The various sense-impressions are the reflex or outcome of their states viewed from the aspect of the various portions differentially affected. Pleasure and Pain are the reflex or outcome of their states viewed from the aspect of efficiency; that is to say, so far as regards their effects on the functions of the organism, considered as a self-regulating machine. Pain is the subjective concomitant of destructive action or insufficient nutrition in any sentient tissue. Pleasure is the subjective concomitant of the normal amount of function in any such tissue. But Pleasure and Pain are only the reflex of the actual state of the nerves, and do not necessarily yield any indications of their future state. Hence, actions which will ultimately yield painful sensations may in their earlier stages be pleasurable, and *vice versâ.* However, in the vast majority of cases, the consensus between the organs, produced by natural selection, is such, that whatever is prejudicial or beneficial to the organism as a whole, is generally painful or pleasurable respectively to the separate organs which it is likely to affect.

Such are, briefly stated, the main principles upon which we must base our system of Æsthetics.

CHAPTER III.

THE DIFFERENTIA OF ÆSTHETICS.

§ 1. *Work and Play.*

HAVING thus arrived at a physiological conception of Pleasure and Pain in general, we have next to consider wherein that class of pleasures and pains known as æsthetic differ from the remainder of their respective genera. And here I can do little else than repeat and expand the definition given by Mr. Herbert Spencer; which, however, I shall try to express in more popular language, besides bringing it into closer connexion with my own plan of treatment.

From the principles laid down in the last chapter, it will naturally follow that the greater part of our pleasures and pains are immediately and directly connected with necessary vital functions. The severest pains are those which result from actual violent dismemberment of any sentient tissue: which action has an obvious importance with reference to the general economy of the body, viewed as a self-conserving mechanism. The greatest physical pleasures are those which result from the normal amount of function in the most essential organic processes; that is, in such processes as are most directly concerned in the maintenance of life both in the individual and in the species. Of these, the two most important are the ingestion of food, that is of fresh energy-yielding matters, which is the necessary condition for maintaining the life of the individual; and the act of procreation, which is the necessary condition for maintaining the life of the species. Hence we might naturally conclude that the processes of eating and drinking and of sexual connexion would be the two greatest physical pleasures of which our nature is capable; and if we take the unsophisticated suffrages of humanity generally, we shall find that these are frankly recognised as such. Furthermore, on mentally running through the list of our chief pleasures and pains, we shall see that they are mostly connected with similar essential life-serving functions.

Now the greater portion of our daily life, taking the average condition of man, is spent in directly or indirectly providing for these necessary physical wants. Work is the ordinary lot of human beings; and to procure food, clothing, shelter, firing, and other necessities of life, is the main object of Work. We may either grow our own food-stuffs, spin and weave our own clothing, build our own hut, and cut our own firewood; or we may fulfil some more specialized function, and so indirectly obtain from others these commodities and services. But in either case the main part of our lives is usually spent in ministering to the wants of our own organisms and those of our offspring, as working machines whose conservation in an efficient state is of prime importance. Every action which conduces to this result may be roughly classed as Work.

The activities thus originated may incidentally produce the pleasures of exercise, though they may equally produce the pains of fatigue. But the immediate pleasure is not the object for which they are undertaken. It is the vital function which they subserve that forms the spring of action, and the gratification, if any, is merely incidental to the pursuit. Work ultimately ministers to the stronger organic pleasures; but it is undertaken for the most part without any immediate agreeable result. There is, however, another class of activities which are entered upon not for any ulterior object, but merely for the gratification which the activity affords. All such comparatively purposeless exercises may be roughly classed as Play. Let us see how these arise.

Every nervous structure in its intervals of repose is perpetually undergoing repair. When repair has continued for a considerable period without fresh discharge, the structure reaches a state of high efficiency, and possesses an unusual quantity of potential energy. Any slight incident energy will then be sufficient to disturb the potential energy stored up in the nervous plexus, so that it will assume the kinetic form. If the consequent activity results in an integration of external matter required by the organism, or in any other life-serving function, the process will belong to that kind of actions which we have roughly classed as Work. But in a certain number of instances the organism will not as a whole require the particular discharge in question, nor will the appropriate object be present; and it will then result in a comparatively purposeless activity, which does not subserve any life-giving process, but which, nevertheless, being a normal manifestation of function in a fully-supplied nervous structure, will have as its subjective concomitant a slight feeling of pleasure. When this pleasure becomes the volitional stimulus to action, the resulting exercise is Play.

Whenever, then, a fully-nourished organ does not obtain its proper amount of function in connexion with the necessary processes of life, there arises a spontaneous tendency for it to exercise itself on any appropriate object which it can discover. This tendency depends upon the existence of leisure (a spare period beyond that required for necessary activity and that required for sleep or repose), which is available for the exercise of activities other than those which contribute to the maintenance of life. Hence arise two classes of impulses, those which give rise to Play, and those which give rise to Art and the Æsthetic Pleasures. What is common to these two classes is their remoteness from life-serving function and their having pleasure alone as their immediate end. We have next to see wherein they differ from one another.

§ 2. *Æsthetic Pleasure differentiated from Play Proper.*

Man, like every other organism, lives perpetually surrounded by an environment. The environment acts upon the organism, and the organism re-acts upon the environment. Hence arise the two fundamental portions of our psychical nature, the passive and the active: a difference incorporated in the nervous system by the sensory and motor fibres and their central organs. Connected with the passive side of our nature, are the organs and faculties of sight, hearing, touch, taste, smell, and organic sensibility generally. Connected with the active side are the muscular system and the nerves which govern it. In this primordial distinction we see the root of the difference which we recognise between Play and the Æsthetic Feelings. The first is active, the second are passive.

When we exercise our limbs and muscles, not for any ulterior life-serving object, but merely for the sake of the pleasure which the exercise affords us, the amusement is called Play. When we similarly exercise our eyes or ears, the resulting pleasure is called an Æsthetic Feeling. In both cases the pleasure is a concomitant of the activity of a well-fed and under-worked organ; but in the latter instance it is on the receptive side, in the former on the re-active. So that Æsthetic Pleasure may be provisionally defined as the subjective concomitant of the normal amount of activity, not directly connected with life-serving function, in the peripheral end-organs of the cerebro-spinal nervous system. What Æsthetic Pain (or rather disagreeable Æsthetic Feeling) may be we shall see hereafter. For the present it will be necessary to turn aside for a moment to a collateral issue.

In the lower senses almost every activity has a direct bearing upon life-giving functions. But in the two higher and specially æsthetic senses, sight and hearing, no activity bears directly upon these functions, and comparatively few even indirectly. Although without sight and hearing we should not be able equally to guide ourselves in search of food, shelter, warmth, and so forth, nor to escape danger, nor to perform many necessary acts; and although we are constantly availing ourselves of these senses for such purposes, which indeed constitute their original intention, yet we incidentally and necessarily see and hear at the same time thousands of sights and sounds which do not so aid us. Now it may be objected that the vast majority of these sights and sounds add no appreciable emotional element to the total of consciousness. This is perfectly true, and the fact throws much light upon the real nature of pleasure and pain. It was noted above that while pleasure is the concomitant of a normal amount of function in sentient tissues, yet for the most part such normal function is not distinctly cognised as pleasurable, but simply remains at the neutral point; because it does not do more than effect the discharge from time to time of the ordinary amount of potential energy which is being perpetually renewed: while all strong pleasures result from the escape of stored-up potential energy which has been hoarded for a considerable period. In the sense of taste, where the organs are only supplied with their appropriate objects at comparatively rare intervals, the nerves are usually so fully nurtured that every stimulant produces a considerable emotional effect, and is distinctly cognised as pleasurable or the reverse. Not till that point of satiety is reached at which we say that the taste is palled or glutted does the feeling become neutral. But in the case of sight and hearing, the organs are so continually undergoing stimulation that very seldom, comparatively, are the nerves nurtured to the extent which gives rise to distinctly pleasurable feelings. For the most part, sights and sounds are only subjects of intellectual discrimination, without yielding appreciable emotional results. Occasionally, however, certain over-fed and under-worked nerves are specially stimulated, and then a faint feeling of pleasure arises; or, on the contrary, certain nerves are called upon to perform an excess of work, beyond their normal functions, and then a faint feeling of pain arises.* And it is just because the eye and the ear are so little connected with vitality that theirs are especially the æsthetic senses. It is the business of Art to combine as many as possible of their pleasurable sensations, and to exclude, so far as lies in its power, all their painful ones; thus producing that synthetic result which we know as the æsthetic thrill.

It may be noted as an illustration that what is thus asserted of the receptive side of our nature is equally true of the active. Most muscular action is neither pleasurable nor painful. Not only is Work proper usually neutral, though it may sometimes prove agreeable to fresh and active nerves and muscles, but even most of our leisure acts—altering the position of our limbs, walking from room to room, taking a constitutional,—are emotionally colourless. But occasionally we consciously undertake certain leisure activities expressly for the pleasure which the exercise will give us; and these leisure activities are what we strictly call

* I say *faint* advisedly, because, as I shall afterwards show, the æsthetic wave is a cumulative effect of many infinitesimal factors.

Play. Similarly when we arrange certain colours or musical notes in certain orders, expressly for the pleasure which their perception will give us, we call the result, Art. So that what Play is to the active faculties, Art and the Æsthetic Pleasures are to the passive.

Finally, just as pleasure in the muscular sense is not necessarily limited to Play, but may incidentally arise from the ordinary exercise of the limbs, so pleasure in the higher senses is not necessarily limited to Art or to consciously-sought æsthetic objects, but may incidentally arise in the contemplation of nature generally.

§ 3. *Further Characteristics of Æsthetic Feelings.*

We have now arrived at some idea of the Æsthetic Feelings. But this idea is incomplete until we have added one or two further limitations. These we can gradually attain by noticing the imperfections of our present conception.

We have seen above that the mass of sights and sounds are emotionally neutral. This is true enough as far as our ordinary consciousness is concerned: and, since pleasures and pains, being facts of consciousness, can only exist when consciously perceived, it is also true absolutely, within certain limits. Yet if we direct our attention to any sight or sound, in order consciously to appraise its æsthetic value, or, in other words, to decide whether it is beautiful or ugly, we shall find that in almost every case it inclines slightly in one direction or the other. The reader can test this for himself by noticing the faces, voices, and clothing of people whom he passes in the street, as well as the buildings and other surroundings on either side. But we also find that while we think of these various *objects* as beautiful or ugly, we do not usually think of the *sensations* they afford us as either pleasant or the reverse. From this apparent paradox, which seems at first sight to contradict our main principle, we can gather two or three additional facts about Æsthetic Feelings.

In the first place, we notice that in ordinary cases the æsthetic quality of objects is so slightly marked that only an exercise of *attention* can bring it definitely into consciousness. (I speak, of course, about the average of humanity; for men of the specially æsthetic temperament instinctively notice these faint impressions without any conscious adjustment of attention.) So we may conclude that in those cases where pleasure is distinctly felt, the total amount of faintly pleasurable sensations must be considerable, and that the effect must be cumulative: which actual observation shows us to be the case. Of this, however, more will be said when we come to examine the senses severally.

Again, since the pleasure or pain afforded by separate elements of sight and sound is so slight, and requires for its perception an exercise of attention, a faculty of our intellectual and volitional nature, it results that in most cases the objects affording the sensations are merely intellectually discriminated as beautiful or ugly, without seeming to any noticeable extent pleasant or painful. Only when the total amount of the emotional wave is very great—as in a fine landscape, a noble painting, a piece of grand music, a lovely woman, on the one hand; or a miserable street, a wretched strumming, a dirty and loathsomely ugly person, on the other—does the emotional element get the better in consciousness of the intellectual. Hence arises the apparent objectivity of beauty and ugliness. The feeling is too little emotional to be referred to a purely internal origin.

And now we see our way clearly to that final principle which forms the ultimate differentia of Æsthetic Feelings. The æsthetically beautiful is that which affords the Maximum of Stimulation with the Minimum of Fatigue or Waste, in processes not directly connected with vital functions. The æsthetically ugly is that which conspicuously fails to do so; which gives little stimulation, or makes excessive and wasteful demands upon certain portions of the organs. But as in either case the emotional element is weak, it is mainly cognised only as an intellectual discrimination. And so we get the idea of the Æsthetic Feelings as something noble and elevated, because they are not distinctly traceable to any life-serving function.

Observe, too, that the æsthetic senses, contrary to the ordinary rule, yield us considerable amounts of appreciable pleasure, but very little appreciable pain. The reason of this is not far to seek. In proportion to the directness of contact with external objects is the liability to violent disruptive actions. Now, the organs of the lower senses, taste and smell, and much more the limbs and muscles generally, are at all times exposed to close contact with destructive agencies in the environment, which give rise to lacerations, burns, bruises, bitter and disagreeable tastes, bad odours, and other similar pains and discomforts. But the eye and ear are specially protected from direct contact with the environment, which they only cognise through the medium of aerial or æthereal undulations. It is true that the nerves of touch distributed to the *conjunctiva*, which lines the eyelid and the outer portion of the eye, are susceptible of ordinary disintegrative action, as when we get a pungent or acid substance under the eyelid: but the optic and auditory nerves proper are so protected as only to be susceptible of stimulation (in normal cases) by their appropriate stimulant. Hence the sole disintegrative action to which they can, under ordinary circumstances, be subjected, is that which arises from excess of the normal activity, not from abnormal destructive excitation. In extreme cases, as when we look at the sun, or hear a loud explosion, the feeling so aroused rises to the intensity of acute pain: but in average cases it is the analogue of that glut or satiety which results in taste or smell from cloying oneself with honey, or with strong perfumes, such as magnolia, stephanotis, and tube-rose. Accordingly, while the normal exercise of the organs yields us pleasure which occasionally rises to the acute pitch, that excessive or inharmonious action which is implied in ugliness does not reach the height of pain.

Note, further, that as the connexion with necessary vital functions decreases, so also does the painfulness of undue stimulation decrease, and sink into mere discomfort, becoming at last that matter of simple intellectual discrimination which marks off the Æsthetic Feelings from the stronger physical pleasures and pains. In organic sensibility the pains felt are violent; in taste, they are rather strong discomforts; in smell they are slighter discomforts; while in sight and hearing they are scarcely more than perceptions of ugliness.

Finally, before we pass on to the next division of our subject, we may notice one last mark of the Æsthetic Feelings which Professor Bain considers as one of their main differentiæ, but which should rather, perhaps, be treated as a property, directly deducible from our general principle—I mean their disinterestedness and freedom from monopoly. As they are only remotely connected with life-serving functions, it follows that they can give pleasure to thousands without detracting from the enjoyment of each. As Professor Bain observes, "The objects of Fine Art, and all objects called æsthetic, are such as may be enjoyed by a great number; some, indeed, are open to the whole human race. They are exempt from the fatal taint of rivalry and contest attaching to other agreeables; they draw men together in mutual sympathy; and are thus eminently social and humanising. A picture or a statue can be seen by millions; a great poem reaches all that understand its language: a fine melody may spread pleasure over the habitable globe. The sunset and the stars are veiled only from the prisoner and the blind."

As a general remark, qualifying each of the special characteristics noticed in this section, it should be added that the æsthetic quality is given to a feeling rather by the concurrence of many such characteristics than by the necessary presence of all or of any particular one. It is consequently somewhat indefinite, and any attempt to define it with strict rigour would be sure either to exclude some true Æsthetic Feelings, or to include some which could hardly claim the title.

§ 4. *Æsthetic Taste.*

At this point in our exposition we are met by a difficulty which has had the effect of making many thinkers reject as impossible all scientific treatment of Æsthetics; the difficulty, namely, arising from that infinite variety of opinion in æsthetic matters which we call Taste. It may plausibly be asked, How can we account for feelings which are seldom or never exactly alike in any two persons? And again it may be objected to the explanation so far foreshadowed that if the perceptions of beauty and ugliness had the physiological origin here sketched out, they ought to be the same in all individuals. Yet we may reasonably conclude *à priori* that, as nervous constitution differs infinitely with regard to minute details in different persons, and as Æsthetic Feelings are the cumulative effect of many infinitesimal physiological factors, the perceptions of beauty and ugliness would differ in various cases to an extent depending upon the structural variations of the nervous system. And this *à priori* inference we find to be borne out by well-known facts.

We will first confine ourselves to the purely sensuous element of Æsthetics, leaving for later consideration the more complex emotional and intellectual factors. And here, to take the most extreme cases first, of course the deaf and the blind cannot possibly experience any kind of Æsthetic Feeling from sounds or visible objects. It may seem absurd to notice such an obvious fact, yet it is worth mentioning as being the ultimate illustration of the principle that differences of perception depend upon differences of structure. Descending to cases of slighter variations, the colour-blind cannot derive the same pleasure as others from judicious combinations of tints; and those utterly destitute of musical ear cannot be gratified or offended by harmony or discord. It is hardly necessary to point out that these differences depend upon abnormal nervous structure. Proceeding to matters of greater detail, all the senses yield us instances of varieties of Taste which are similarly referable to slight morphological peculiarities. In the gustatory sense everybody has his own likes and dislikes. Children, with delicate organs and nervous centres not blunted by use, are offended by curry, mustard, cayenne, and similar pungent condiments; while those adults whose palate is spoilt require such violent stimulants in order to arouse jaded sensation. Persons of strong digestion and healthy livers enjoy butter, oil, fat, and rich dishes; whereas those of opposite diathesis are disgusted by them, owing to the sympathy which exists between the stomach and the entrance of the alimentary canal. Like varieties are found in the sense of smell. Musk, which is a pleasing stimulant to coarse or voluptuous natures, is an overpowering odour to the delicately or austerely constituted. Some people are unable to bear the perfume of strongly-scented flowers, such as jasmine: others are not offended even by caviare, ambergris, or patchouli. In the sense of hearing, savages and children, whose nerves are fresh and strong, are pleased by the violent stimulation of beating a tom-tom or a tin kettle, shouting an unvaried note, or blowing a penny whistle: while most civilised adults are annoyed by such noises, and valetudinarians cannot endure the creaking of a door or the noise of wind round the eaves. Monotony, which obviously makes excessive demands upon certain nervous structures, is intensely disagreeable to the musically cultivated, but seems rather pleasing to the less discriminative nervous centres of the utterly untutored ear. In a less degree of antithesis (involving certain complex emotional factors), the audience at a classical concert are gratified by the complex harmony of Bach's fugues; while the public of a music-hall admire a chorus of Offenbach, and the street boys derive greater pleasure from the rollicking and boisterous melody of a comic song. In sight (omitting the phenomena of long and short sight, whose effects are rather intellectual than emotional) the vulgar are pleased by great masses of colour, especially red, orange, and purple, which give their coarse nervous organisation the requisite stimulus: the refined, with nerves of less calibre but greater discriminativeness, require delicate combinations of complementaries, and prefer neutral tints to the glare of primary hues. Children and savages love to dress in all the colours of the rainbow; a Parisian costume is rather noticeable for its graceful outline, its rich trimmings, and the effects of harmony or contrast in its arrangement. Compare an Egyptian painting, staring in red, green, and yellow, with a water-colour by David Cox; or the scarlet and blue porcelain figures in a tap-room with Gibson's tinted Venus; and recollect that each has its own circle of admirers. So that everywhere we see minor varieties of structure—central or peripheral—entailing minor variations in Æsthetic Feeling, of which we ordinarily speak as Taste.

If we examine these various cases, how do we find them reconcilable with the notion of a science of Æsthetics? Simply thus.—In spite of the minor variations here described, the vast majority of feelings are pleasurable or painful, as the case may be, to the vast majority of men alike. With every average individual, sweets are agreeable and bitters disagreeable; fresh meat allures and putrescent meat repels; perfumes are pleasant and stenches noisome: notwithstanding certain slight variations in certain unimportant details. And similarly with sights and sounds: setting aside very abnormal cases, all alike enjoy the sunset and the rainbow, butterflies and flowers, mountains and waterfalls, the song of birds and simple melodies; though by no means all equally with one another. Were it not so, Art, which trades upon these common tastes, would be impossible. But just as the confectioner and the perfumer can judge what is likely to please the palate and the nose of their customers, so the artist can discover what will please the taste of his public.* Nay, even such trades as those of the dyer, the house-painter, and the stone-cutter point to the same truth; for every one of the operations which they perform is intended simply to enhance the beauty of the goods in which they deal. It will be seen hereafter (indeed it is clear enough to any one who chooses to run through the various cases for himself) that in the

* A qualification of this statement is given on page 49.

civilised state there is scarcely a manufactured article in daily use on which some attempt is not made to give æsthetic additions. Let the reader cast his eye about his room and notice the pattern and colours of the wall-paper, the carpet, and the hearth-rug; the mouldings of the cornice, the fender, and the gas-hangings; the polish on the chairs, the table, and the coal-scuttle; the gilding on the curtain-rings, the mirror, the binding of the books; the very bevelling on the doors, the mantel-piece, and the wainscot; and he will see that every one of them has a decorative purpose. I omit the pictures, the vases, the statuettes, the Japanese fans, which are there for ornament alone, and the piano, which subserves a purely æsthetic function; but if the reader merely examines the grate and the fire-irons, he will see how universally even in the most utilitarian articles care is taken to gratify the æsthetic sentiment. The veriest savage carves a grotesque head upon his club, and adorns his calabash with circles and crosses. Now all that any science need primarily account for is the normal and usual phenomena of its subject-matter; when those are fully understood, it may pass on to the abnormal and unusual. Our first object must be, not to explain the Æsthetic Feelings of a Raphael, a Mozart, or a Milton, but those of the average human being with whom we come in daily contact. Indeed, it seems to me that one of the greatest errors in disquisitions on Æsthetics is this, that they take for the most part only the very highest developments of the sentiment, and endeavour to explain them without previous reference to the simpler cases. I shall be satisfied, on the other hand, if I can account physiologically for the common pleasure in bright coloured objects, elementary paintings, easy melodies, and popular poetry: only touching slightly upon the more involved phenomena of kindred origin.

To apply a metaphor drawn from another science, Taste may be regarded as the *personal equation* of Æsthetics, for which allowance must in each case be made, but which does not detract from the objective truth of the general result. Only, in Æsthetics, where we are dealing with phenomena of the nervous system itself, the personal equation rises into such great importance as to form one of the main departments of the subject. So we must always endeavour to account, not merely for the most usual form of Taste, but also for the structural peculiarities which give rise to the principal variations. And especially must we do so in treating of those varieties which differentiate the artistically-minded few from the inartistic masses.

Again, we have only looked so far at the sensuous or presentative elements of Æsthetic Feeling. But when we remember that it includes, beside, a vast body of emotional and intellectual—that is, representative—elements, the difficulty of accounting for these varieties in Taste is still further decreased. As men and women differ infinitely in emotions and intellect, they must differ infinitely in their appreciation of that which calls up emotional and intellectual activities of various orders in various combinations. We cannot expect a child or a savage to admire the poetry of Wordsworth, the landscapes of Turner, the sonatas of

Beethoven, the duomo of Milan. Yet even here we see this community of feeling, that what is at once simple and beautiful is pleasing to the highest and lowest intelligences alike:—instance a daisy or a butterfly, an old English melody, or a Homeric ballad. And here, too, as before, we need only account for those feelings which are most common and universal, knowing that the special and higher ones are merely more complicated and more representative combinations of the same elements.

Nor must we suppose, because Æsthetic Feelings are simply relative to the nervous organisation of the individual, that an absolute æsthetic standard is impossible, and that good and bad Taste are mere matters of convention. On the contrary, it follows from what has been said above that bad Taste is the concomitant of a coarse and indiscriminative nervous organisation, an untrained attention, a low emotional nature, and an imperfect intelligence; while good Taste is the progressive product of progressing fineness and discrimination in the nerves, educated attention, high and noble emotional constitution, and increasing intellectual faculties. Though it is obviously impossible for us at our present point of development, confessedly imperfect, to set up a final and absolute standard of Taste, we are yet bound to accept as a relative and temporary standard, the judgment of the finest-nurtured and most discriminative, the purest and most cultivated of our contemporaries, who have paid the greatest attention to æsthetic perceptions; assured that while it may fall far short of absolute perfection, it will at any rate be far truer and higher than that of the masses. If we fail to agree with them, while we recognise the fact as final, we must attribute it to the imperfection of our own sensuous and emotional nature, or of our artistic education. At the same time we must not attempt to impose such a standard upon ourselves or others faster than our development enables us to receive it. We cannot transmute our Tastes; we can only educate them. It may have appeared a hard saying when I remarked just now that the artist knows what will please his public: it seemed, and justly seemed, a degradation to the highest artist, whose Taste must always be a little in advance of that of his patrons. But the explanation is simple. There are artists for every class of public, from the most cultured to the vulgarest, and they each know what their public requires. The highest, who work up to the standard of their own Taste, usually gain little recognition during their life-time. But the Taste which they have educated gains them at last a late or a posthumous recognition; while the little artist of the day passes away and is forgotten. The works of the highest Art, like the works of the highest Intellect, necessarily appeal to a very limited audience.

We may briefly sum up the contents of this section in two common adages. While it is true that "de gustibus non est disputandum," it is eminently untrue that "there's no accounting for Tastes."

§ 5. *Æsthetic Education.*

If Æsthetic Feelings depend, as has been said, upon our nervous constitution,—sensuous, emotional, intellectual,—

how can there be such a thing as the Education of Taste?

In answering this question we must first premise that here, as elsewhere, the range of Education is comparatively limited. All that it can ever effect is to *educe* the existing faculties, not to *produce* new ones. As in the intellect we can make the student employ all the powers he possesses, and strengthen them by employment, but cannot lead him up beyond the limit which his cerebral structure lays upon his intelligence: so in Æsthetics, we can teach ourselves to observe every faint wave of pleasure or pain, every delicate thrill of harmony, every minute twinge of discord, which our nervous organisation renders us capable of perceiving, but we can never get beyond this natural barrier, or transcend our own organic capacities. To employ the extreme illustration used above, the colour-blind cannot possibly be taught to enjoy dainty contrasts of tint, nor the note-deaf to be offended at musical discords. In every department the aim of Education should be so to train each individual that he may use to the best advantage the organism which heredity and circumstances have given him. More than this it cannot possibly effect.

Fully allowing this restriction, we find that Taste may be to a considerable extent educated within the possible limits. There are two ways in which this can be done. The first is by the exercise of Attention, the second by the growth of new intellectual and emotional Associations. We will briefly examine each in order.

As Æsthetic Feelings are composed of very faint impressions of pleasure and pain, seldom rising conspicuously into the foreground of consciousness, and only for the most part intellectually cognised, it follows that their recognition must greatly depend upon the amount of Attention bestowed on them. Other things being equal as to original endowment, we derive pleasure and discomfort from our æsthetic environment, in proportion as we are surrounded from childhood upward by beautiful objects, and as we are taught (or teach ourselves) consciously to compare the effects of combination, symmetry, and contrast. Harmonies and discords, which at first escaped our notice, become gradually more and more apparent. Lights and shades, undertones and beats, disregarded by the ordinary eye and ear, are watched for and observed by the cultivated. To the untrained spectator, a tree is a mass of unbroken green, an egg is a surface of pure white; to the artistic vision they are both infinitely complicated fields of varying hues. While the common mind, in which the intellectual side is uppermost, translates the outward impression too rapidly into the reality which it symbolises,—interprets the sensations instead of observing them;—the æsthetic mind, in which the emotional side is uppermost, dwells rather upon the actual impression received, in all the minuteness of its slightest detail. And so the highest artist, in his very fidelity to nature, lays himself open in the mind of the vulgar to the charge of imagining or inventing the faint effects of colour which *he* has the skill and the care to perceive, but which *they* neither do see, can see, nor take the trouble to see.

But besides the Education which is the result of attention, there is also an Education which is the result of Association, intellectual and emotional. In its simplest form this consists in the formation of standards of reference. When we first see mountains or waterfalls, we are unable to judge rightly of them, because we have nothing with which to make a comparison. But after we have seen several of each class, we can compare the height, the contour, the colouring of the one, the volume, the foam, the leap of the other. As Mr. Herbert Spencer truly says, every cognition is a recognition. And in the very act of comparison there arises a pleasure, due to the active exercise of the intellectual organs. We can classify waterfalls (to take a concrete example) into those which, like Gavarnie, the Staubbach, and the Grey Mare's Tail, leap headlong from a precipice in a thin thread of spray; those which, like Montmorenci, Foyers, and Tivoli, come down in an unbroken sheet of foam; those which, like Niagara and Schaffhausen, pour majestically over a ledge in a broad cataract; and those which, like Ste. Anne, the Giesbach, and the Swallow Fall, are broken into small cascades, or widen out toward their base into the shape of an open fan. As we gaze at the particular fall before us, it fits itself naturally into one or other of these classes, and is mentally compared in a thousand points of detail with various similar instances seen before. Moreover, we thus arrive at a clearer view of the points in the object which call for our admiration. Persons who as children have been familiar with the view of Niagara do not fully realise its stupendous mass and force. But when such a person, gifted with average æsthetic sensibility, travels elsewhere, visits other famous cataracts, and familiarises himself with their volume, he is astonished, on returning once more to Niagara, to see how vastly it has grown in sublimity and beauty.*

This formation of standards of reference is, as noted above, the simplest instance of Education by Association. Art supplies us with more complex cases. We grow at last to love the special touch of our favourite masters, and the recognition of their style, or of some delicate imitation of it in particular points, gives rise to an emotional thrill of familiarity. In any modern composition a dash of Claude or of Vandyke, a reminiscence of Mendelssohn, a Dantesque or Virgilian touch, comes back to us with a glow of delight. Tennyson's "faint Homeric echoes," or occasional Miltonic ring, carry with them clustered memories of older poets. The thoroughly æsthetic mind is stored with such scraps of recollection, and projects them even into its appreciation of nature. A meadow scene is admired because it is just what Cuyp would have loved to paint; a bit of still life is in the very style of Sneyders; a head and figure are Reynolds himself; a half-length in the gloom is a perfect Rembrandt. Architecture affords perhaps the best instance of the increase of discrimination which comes with increase of knowledge. Our first childish, half-unconscious admiration of a large and ornamented building, grows at last into the conscious

* It is at once amusing and instructive for the English reader to find "Mark Twain" judging the scenery of Europe and the East with the lakes and mountains of Colorado and Nevada for his standard of reference.

critical pleasure derived from a perfect example of any particular style, age, or nation,—the Parthenon, the Palace of Diocletian, the façade of Cologne, the lantern of St. Ouen; or into the conscious critical disgust at a mongrel and meaningless fabric,—the Brighton Pavilion, the Oxford Museum, the Capitol at Washington, the Albert Memorial. But these effects of Association will have to be more fully discussed in the later chapters of this work, and may be left for the present with such brief notice as they have already received.

§ 6. *Total Effect of the Æsthetic Environment on Happiness.*

To guard against misapprehension, it may be well here to say a few words upon the relation to Happiness of Æsthetic Feelings in the gross. I have mentioned above that they afford us on the whole comparatively slight amounts of pleasure, while, on the other hand, contrary to the general rule, they are capable of yielding a greater proportion of pleasure than of pain. Both these statements need a little qualification, more for the sake of disarming criticism than of adding very largely to our views upon the subject.

The remark that Æsthetic Feelings afford comparatively slight amounts of pleasure must of course be understood as referring to each separate element regarded in isolation. Even in masses, they require a comparatively free field to make any great impression. They cannot be greatly enjoyed in sickness, poverty, or depressed conditions of mind. But when they enter largely into the current of a life free from serious pains, difficulties, or vexations, they may form a considerable element in Happiness. To live in a noble building, standing amid beautiful grounds, surrounded by objects of fine art, which lend an æsthetic charm to even the commonest processes of daily life, such as eating and drinking, is of course the final crown of beauty to an existence otherwise free from urgent cares and the sordid shifts of poverty. Not only does it make life happier, but it makes it something brighter, higher, and more ethereal. Even to move for a short time in such surroundings sheds a grace about one's being for the moment which is remembered long after with pleasure. And to those who necessarily lead a life of hard work or drudgery, the brief annual escape to Switzerland or the Lakes, to the sea or the green fields, as each can afford, is looked forward to, and looked back upon, as the greatest pleasure of the year, a feast for eyes and ears, lungs and muscles. Yet in each case it is worth while to remember that many other feelings besides the æsthetic are involved in this complex total; such as the delights of freedom, of power, of pride, of fresh air and muscular exercise, of novelty and variety, and of mental rest. On the whole, we may safely say that æsthetic pleasure in the mass is of great importance as complementary, but requires a basis of physical and mental well-being before it can become to any great extent an element of Happiness.

With regard to the second statement, that Æsthetic Feelings yield us a greater proportion of pleasure than of pain, it will be well to add that this is only true in the average of cases; an exceptional instance occasionally occurs where the æsthetic environment is so utterly squalid and miserable as to give rise to a continuous state of discomfort almost amounting to positive pain. Although ugliness is for the most part only intellectually cognised as such, without emotional effect, yet if persons accustomed to ordinarily beautiful surroundings are suddenly transported into the midst of peculiarly ugly circumstances, they discover that the change is capable of producing a very genuine feeling of distress and misery. No inhabitant of a West End square would enjoy life in the Seven Dials. Exiles to our tropical dependencies find in many cases that the filthy and dilapidated streets—the dirty, ragged, and diseased condition of the population—the bare and inartistic homes—the total want of æsthetic taste, and of all care for beauty in the concerns of every-day life,—all affect them with a disgust which actually preys upon the spirits. Of course here, too, we must allow for intellectual and emotional disturbances as well, such as the low standard of education and intelligence in the society with which one must mix; or the moral repugnance at European insolence, African degradation, and Mongolian ethical filthiness; beside taking into account the purely physical influence of climate in depressing the tone of the nervous system.*

* This last-named cause, besides making ugliness more than usually ugly (because any excessive demand upon the nerves is most painful when they ar weakest), almost totally deprives us of the power of enjoying beauty, eve when present. I have seen views in the tropics in which I could intellectually recognise all the elements of beauty, so that I gave in a verbal adhesion to the proposition that they were lovely, while at the same time they utterly

But after all allowances made, it yet remains an indisputable fact that in such exceptional circumstances the æsthetically ugly nature of our surroundings does contribute in a very appreciable degree towards rendering life dull and gloomy. Persons in such a case are astonished to find how large a portion of their happiness has consisted, unconsciously to themselves, of Æsthetic Pleasures. This is often shown by the attempt which is spasmodically made under such conditions by many Europeans, who are elsewhere comparatively careless about their personal environment, to make home and home life as beautiful as possible with flowers, pictures, graceful furniture, and musical instruments; and having attained to this somewhat selfish isolation, to keep as far as may be within the domestic circle, and never unnecessarily encounter the squalid sights without. Yet these exceptional instances only occur where an individual whose æsthetic taste has been highly cultivated in one set of circumstances is removed into a new environment for which he is not fitted. They cannot be held to militate against the general truth that the Æsthetic Feelings differ from the majority of our faculties in yielding us comparatively much pleasure and comparatively little pain.

failed to produce in me the faintest thrill of pleasure. Photographs of the same places, seen now under an English sky and an English nervous diathesis, strike me as exquisitely beautiful.

CHAPTER IV

THE LOWER SENSES.

§ 1. *The Chemical Sensibility of the Skin.*

OUR main concern in the present work will be with the two higher and specially æsthetic senses, those of Sight and Hearing. But it will assist us greatly in comprehending the phenomena of these if we first glance briefly at the lower senses of Taste and Smell, as well as at the intermediate one of Touch. We shall thus bridge over the gulf which intervenes between the purely organic pleasures and pains, and those of the æsthetic class, which might otherwise appear too wide a gap for a single leap. Moreover, as sensations of Taste and Smell, in their ideal form, enter considerably into the structure of Poetry, the highest of the æsthetic arts, it will be necessary to examine them shortly here in the actuality, in order that we may afterwards account for their pleasurable or painful nature in the representation. And it will accordingly be desirable, first, to look a little at the general sensibility of the body which underlies all these special forms, and of which they are only highly-differentiated varieties.

The reader must remember throughout that we have to

deal with these various senses chiefly from the point of view of pleasure and pain, and are not at all concerned with the purely intellectual problem of discrimination, which occupies the whole attention in most treatises on the senses, whether physiological or psychological. He must therefore be prepared to find many familiar facts omitted, and many comparatively slight manifestations brought into prominence, according as they do or do not bear upon the purely emotional question.

There are five ways in which external agencies can affect the body. The *first* is by mechanical action, and the *second* by heat, for the perception of which we are provided with a network of nerves over the whole surface. The *third* mode is by chemical action, for which we possess the special sense-organs of Taste and Smell. The *fourth* is by the impact of æthereal or aerial undulations, which we cognise through the organs of Sight and Hearing. The *fifth* is by electrical action, which occurs so seldom in nature that we have no special organ for its perception. It is with the third class of organs, those which are affected by chemical action, that we must first deal. As illustrative of these, we must begin by looking at certain analogous phenomena in the general sensibility of the skin.

The human skin consists of three membranes, the epidermis, the mucous layer, and the dermis or true skin. The first-named tissue is completely devoid of blood and nerves, and is of course totally insentient. The other layers are supplied with sensory nerves, whose principal terminations are not simple, but consist of a central body and numerous surrounding convolutions, which finally lose themselves in its mass. These end-organs are called tactile corpuscles, and are considered to be the instruments of the sense of Touch. Now, the ordinary method of stimulating these nerves is by mechanical pressure; but there is also another and rarer method, when particles of highly penetrative substances are absorbed through the epidermis, and act chemically upon the sentient tissues beneath. Cases of this latter sort must necessarily depend upon the chemical character of the substances and the thickness or other peculiarities of the epidermis in the part affected. Let us examine a few in order.

Caustic substances and corrosive acids actually destroy the tissues by their violent chemical action. Take as instances caustic potash, and nitric or sulphuric acid. These, however, act upon the nervous structures only after destroying the superjacent epidermis. In other cases the substance penetrates the outer skin, and sets up actions in the underlying tissues. A common illustration will be found in the operation of a mustard plaster, and a still stronger one in that of a cantharides blister. Capsicums, cut in two and laid upon the skin, cause inflammation, accompanied by a stinging pain. In fact most pungent substances act upon the skin in the same manner as upon the tongue, though to a less degree. Again, acids generally, when beyond a certain strength, cause a slight tingling sensation when applied to the body: vinegar does so very noticeably. Alkalies usually warp the part to which they are applied. Ammonia, too, is rapidly absorbed through the skin, and gives rise to a considerable amount of smarting. Alcoholic spirits, rubbed into thin-skinned parts, set up a faint tingling. In short, most highly diffusible and chemically-active substances, when placed upon the skin, are absorbed into the tissues, and there give rise to chemical changes. When these changes are slight in character, they are perhaps faintly pleasurable (as stimulation) or else neutral; when they reach a destructive point, they are painful and occcasionally rise to the acute pitch.

Moreover, this liability to be chemically affected is greater in some parts of the body than in others, varying chiefly as the thickness of the epidermis. It is least on the heel and the palm of the hand; greatest on the cheek, neck, and abdomen. Where the epidermis is modified and passes into the thinner epithelial membranes, the liability to excitement in this manner is very great indeed. All pungent substances placed upon such structures (for example, the inner surface of the eyelids) act upon them even more violently than upon the tongue, though the resulting feeling is cognised chiefly as pain, without much intellectual discrimination. Pepper or vinegar, under such circumstances, give rise to a very similar smart. At any rate, we see throughout that sensibility to chemical action is a common property of sentient tissues, but that it is most conspicuous where the thinnest layers of insentient tissue intervene between the nerves and the substance which acts upon them.

Now the organs of Taste and Smell are surfaces copiously

supplied with bundles of nerves, concentrated in large numbers on a comparatively small area, their terminations being naked points in a very modified membrane, so as to be unusually exposed and yield in consequence unusually large volumes of this general chemical sensibility. And they are placed at the entrance of the alimentary and respiratory canals, where they act as discriminative of the foodstuffs or gases taken into the body, and yield, by the pleasure or pain which they give, some indication of their probable effect on the system as a whole.

But before we go on to examine them in detail, it will be well to explain one point to which allusion has been made above. The feelings aroused in the mouth or nose by the bodies mentioned in the preceding paragraphs differ from the chemical sensibility of the skin, in that they are distinctively cognised as tastes and smells. This difference depends upon a general principle of our subjectivity which is known as *the law of specific energies.* According to this principle, each separate nerve and its connected centre are only capable of yielding us a single kind of sensation, whatever may be the stimulant employed. For example, the optic nerve, whether cut, pressed, galvanised, or injured, yields a sensation of light; the auditory similarly yields sounds; and the gustatory, tastes. So, too, separate portions of each main trunk yield special qualities of sensation: thus certain fibres of the optic nerve are considered to afford only the sensation of red, while others give us that of green; and in the same manner certain auditory fibres are supposed to be appropriated to notes of a particular pitch. Accordingly, we must suppose that subjective differences depend, not on the stimulus applied, but on the portion of the central organs affected. This law we must provisionally take for granted, leaving its further exemplification for the detailed account of the various senses.

§ 2. *Taste.*

The organ of Taste is the tongue, with which may perhaps be associated the palate. Its mucous membrane is abundantly supplied with nervous papillæ, of different kinds, and connected with different trunk nerves. The terminals lie in little goblet-shaped depressions, so that all substances which are to affect them must be in solution; for which purpose the mouth is furnished with a dissolving liquid, the saliva. Sapid bodies are moistened by the saliva, and affect the terminals through the very delicate cell-membrane alone. Only crystalloids are sapid, colloids not possessing the necessary diffusibility. Very little is known as to the physiology of Taste, and hence we shall be driven to a somewhat conjectural treatment of this sense.

The tongue has been conveniently divided by Professor Bain, so far as its sensibility is concerned, into three regions. The first is that in which nerves of touch predominate; the second is that supplied with nerves of taste proper; and the third is that whose nerves are in close sympathy with the stomach. Each of these requires separate treatment.*

The nerves of touch distributed to the tongue belong to

* I adopt Professor Bain's division and localization only after a series of experimental tests, which I hope to detail at some other opportunity.

the lingual branch of the Fifth Cerebral Pair, and are most closely concentrated on its upper extremity. These are the nerves which bear the greatest analogy in their action to the general chemical sensibility of the body. Whatever gives rise to a sensation of that order when placed upon the skin, gives rise to a sensation of tactual Taste when placed upon the tip of the tongue. But the lingual sensation differs in two respects from the dermal; in the first place it is more acute, and in the second it is more discriminative. The first peculiarity is doubtless due to the greater exposure of the nerves, the second to their being differentially assigned to different stimulants, and terminating in different percipient centres. The special Tastes which we thus distinguish are the pungent, the astringent, the alkaline, the acid, and the saline.

Taking the various stimulants already mentioned as giving rise to chemical sensations in the tissues at large, we may notice that caustic substances and corrosive acids, which destroy the organic structures generally, act in precisely the same manner upon the tongue. Accordingly, we find that they yield us a feeling of pain alone, not of Taste: that is, they are only emotionally cognised, not intellectually discriminated. Sulphuric acid, which, if greatly diluted, can be *tasted*, can only be said, when a drop is placed in the pure state upon the tongue, to *burn*. Passing on to those substances which, instead of destroying the whole mucous membrane, only act upon the nerve-terminations; we all know that mustard produces the same sort of effect, though more instantaneously, upon the tongue as upon the skin generally. Similarly with capsicums, cayenne, pepper, cress, and other pungent bodies. The slight tingling which accompanies hypodermal absorption of acids, is more distinctly cognised in the tongue as sourness. Alkalies act upon the mouth in the same warping manner as upon the skin, the main difference being one of greater distinctness. Ammonia bites the palate with a sharpness extremely akin to its effect on the nose and the body. Alcoholic spirits burn the mouth, very much as they burn the inner surface of the eyelid. So that we see reason everywhere for regarding the special chemical sensibility of the lingual nerve as an intensified modification of the general chemical sensibility of the body at large.

The stimulations thus effected are in the main and in unsophisticated cases almost purely painful: and we know by their action upon other tissues that they are of a destructive character. A very small amount of mustard or pepper might perhaps originally be agreeable as a stimulant; but, I believe, they are distasteful, even in the minutest quantities, to the delicate organs of infants. Later on, as the natural irritability of the fibres and nerve-centres is blunted by use, we come gradually to require these more violent excitations, in order to arouse sensation at all. We begin with small quantities of mustard and pepper; we progress soon to water-cress and radishes; at last we go on to curries and mulligatawny; and if we have ruined our taste with these, we finally require the fierce stimulation of pungent sauces, red peppers, and devilled meats. Similarly with drinks. Our first liking for milk passes into a taste for beer and claret; thence we progress to sherry and madeira; and when these cease sufficiently to bite the blunted sense, we may descend at last to neat spirits, absinthe, and American mixtures.

But in all such cases it should be noticed that, originally at least, we employ such acid and pungent substances only as *condiments;* that is, in small quantities to add piquancy to what in itself lacks flavour. No one of them can be eaten alone. They are not food, they are accompaniments to food. We use vinegar merely as a dressing for beet-root, salad, or pickled salmon; we put a fragment of chili in our soup; and we never dream of tossing off a tumblerful of Worcestershire sauce. Even in such cases as radishes and water-cress, the pungency is only incidental, the main attraction being the freshness, coolness, and delicacy of the vegetable: when they grow old, stringy, and fiery, or lose their crispness by keeping, we reject them. Alcohol is endured for the sake of its cordial effects, and of the flavours by which it is disguised: in proportion as it is pure it becomes distasteful. Everybody at once recognises that the taste which cannot be satisfied except by red-hot sauces and burning curries is a morbid and perverted one. A judicious palate prefers mustard in the softened form which French manufacturers give it, and uses pungent stimulants sparingly. In every case a point is at last reached where the action ceases to be mere stimulation, and becomes destructive or disintegrative. That point, in each individual instance, forms, of course, the boundary between simple pungency and pain. Nothing shows more clearly the naturally disintegrative nature of the stimulation than the fact that no pleasurable excitement passes more readily or more habitually into pain. An overdose of condiments which brings tears into our eyes is one of our most familiar experiences.

The reason for this mechanism is clear enough. We must remember that the theory of evolution, while it rejects the idea of design, yet, by substituting for it the notion of natural selection, leaves most teleological explanations exactly where they were.* The consensus which is slowly produced between the different portions of an organism is the necessary condition of that organism's survival. In the highest species we must expect to see this consensus carried out in great detail; and the sense of Taste in man supplies us, in all three of its divisions, with an excellent example of such minute provision. The nature of the external bodies integrated by the organism being of prime importance, we naturally find at the entrance of the alimentary canal a system of highly discriminative nervous structures, in harmony as to pleasure and pain with the organism generally. Confining ourselves to the portion immediately under investigation we see that the entrance of the oral cavity is provided with a specially thin membrane, so as to yield us immediate information concerning the presence of those caustic or corrosive substances which instantaneously and energetically attack the tissues. Next, the tip of the tongue is so constituted as to be specially sensitive to small

* An exception must be made for those structures which, like the fœtal teeth of whales and the caudal vertebræ of man, are mere obsolescent relics of a once useful mechanism.

quantities of pungent, acid, or alkaline bodies, which, if swallowed in any great amount, would produce disastrous results upon the stomach and intestines. It consequently informs us of the presence of these, and acts as a natural check against our swallowing them in larger quantities or more concentrated forms than the system can easily endure. And in infancy, when even very slight amounts might prove dangerous, it prompts us energetically and entirely to reject them. But if the substance which it is proposed to integrate proves pleasant or neutral to this tactual region of the mouth, it is passed on for the further verdict of the purely gustatory nerves, and is finally entrusted to the portion of the organ of Taste in sympathy with the stomach; after successfully passing all which, it is handed over to the automatic process of swallowing, with a considerable probability of proving uninjurious to the digestive organs. To the second of these regions we may now proceed.

The sense of Taste proper is located in the middle of the tongue. Its nerves are twigs of the glosso-pharyngeal. It is by means of these, apparently, that we are sensible of those special Tastes called *sweet* and *bitter*. The name "Taste" ought in strictness be limited to them, as those lingual sensations which we have hitherto considered are rather tactual than gustatory; while for the third class, in sympathy with the stomach, Professor Bain has proposed the convenient terms "relish" and "disgust." It is to be regretted that we have not some more general name under which the three classes might be subsumed.

Sweet and bitter Tastes form the real crux of the present

question. The sensations with which we have hitherto dealt proved on examination to be mere intensified varieties of the ordinary chemical sensibility; but this is not exactly the case with sweet and bitter Tastes. Sugar and aloes if placed upon the skin in solution do not produce any sensation beyond that of touch-proper. Not even when applied to the thinner epithelial membranes do they yield any distinctive manifestation. Hence we must conclude that the pure gustatory nerve has been specially modified in the course of our development so as to be chemically stimulated by certain absorbed substances which do not equally affect the other nerves. We must also infer, by analogy with other cases, that the modification is of such a nature as to make the nerve be healthily stimulated by those objects which are called sweet, and destructively attacked by those objects which are called bitter. In short, I would propose that the doctrine of specific energies, which has hitherto been applied to intellectual discrimination alone, should be extended to emotional phenomena as well. While the specific pain of the eye is called "dazzling," and that of the ear "deafening," the specific pain of the tactual Taste is a *pungent smart*, and the specific pleasures and pains of the gustatory nerve are known as *sweets* and *bitters*, or *relishes* and *disgusts*, respectively, according to the fibres affected. This explanation would account for the singular variety of chemical constitution in sweet and bitter objects. The sole community between them would be the power of normally or excessively stimulating certain gustatory fibres; a power which might easily be possessed by the most different bodies. That sweet tastes are normally stimulative is evidenced by the fact that no concentration of sweetness ever becomes painful; the only disagreeable feeling that can result from them being the fatigue of excessive excitation, which we call being cloyed; and even this is very slowly induced. That bitter tastes are actively destructive is evidenced by the fact that they are not pleasant, as mere stimulation, even in the minutest quantities: whence we may conclude that their action is instantaneously disintegrative, since whenever there is a sufficient amount of the sapid body to be perceived at all, it is perceived as unpleasant: or, to put the same proposition in objective instead of subjective terms, wherever there is a particle of the body large enough to affect the nerves at all, it affects them in a destructive manner. Although we cannot yet account chemically and physiologically for the mode of operation in either case, yet we can easily see why, in the gradual formation of the consensus between the organs, a modification which would produce this effect must naturally arise.

Almost all the vegetable productions which enter largely into the food of man, especially in the uncivilized state, are characterized by the presence of sugar in greater or less quantities. Still more is this the case with those tubers, fruits, and succulent portions of plants, which are fitted for the use of the Quadrumana generally. Hence the fact that a natural substance contains sugar becomes in the unsophisticated state a rough test of its desirability as food to a mainly herbivorous race; and we might consequently expect that there would be developed in them, at the entrance to the alimentary canal, a nervous structure which would be agreeably stimulated by sugar, and so give an inducement to the act of swallowing substances which contained it. Just such a nervous structure actually exists; and moreover the natural sustenance provided for the infant, milk, possesses a sweet taste, and so forms an incentive to the act of sucking. Starch, indeed, would have proved an equally good rough test; but then starch does not possess the diffusibility of sugar, into which it passes after the process of salivation. Moreover, sugar is characterized in a remarkable degree by the power of stimulating the flow of saliva, and thus mechanically facilitating the act of swallowing: while, on the contrary, substances which did not contain it would mostly fail to rouse the saliva, and so be rejected as dry and unsavoury.

On the other hand, if we look at the majority of bitter substances, we shall see that, in the midst of a perplexing variety of chemical constitution, they agree very largely in a single characteristic, that of being destructive or injurious to life when swallowed. Those vegetable alkaloids which, like quinine and strychnia, are intensely bitter, are also violent nervous irritants; and though in certain morbid states of body they may be taken with advantage in small quantities as tonics, yet they are when eaten at all plentifully for the most part so highly injurious as to belong to that class of destructive bodies known as poisons. Now what we call their tonic or irritant property is in reality a power of exciting strong or excessive action in the nervous centres, which they reach in small quantities and a highly diluted form, through the blood: accordingly, we cannot be surprised that they should exercise a powerful destructive action on the specially unstable nerve-terminations of the tongue, on which they are placed in comparatively large quantities, and in a highly concentrated form. Again, the bitter principle of colocynth, and of the seeds and pulps of many gourds and melons, is a drastic purgative. The bitter end of cucumber is similarly poisonous. Rhubarb and aloes are commonly known as strong aperients. Decaying apples contain a bitter and injurious substance known as maloïl. Lactucin, the compound which imparts to lettuce stalks their unpleasant taste, is a narcotic. Wormwood, orange rind, chesnut and walnut shells, contain other bitter and injurious principles. But perhaps the most common of all these bodies is that known as amygdalin, the sapid principle of bitter almonds, found also in peach and plumstones, apple pippins, and many other fruits. This, under the influence of ferments, splits up into various components, of which prussic acid is one. Hence it will be observed that poisonous bitters constantly occur in close conjunction with articles of food, and especially with some which form the usual diet of the Quadrumana. So that we might expect the same natural selection which aided the development of a taste for sugar to aid the development of a converse affection of the tongue by the common vegetable poisons. Such a provision is especially necessary, as the dangerous substance is often so closely conjoined with the ordinary food. This last consideration helps to account for the unpleasantness of bitter tastes even in the smallest amounts.

Furthermore, we see here an instance of that wider consensus which is necessary between the whole fauna and flora in order that animal and vegetable life may each be kept up. While it is often advantageous to the plant that its seed should be swallowed by animals and so dispersed, or deposited by them in a nourishing matrix of their excreta, it is disadvantageous in the highest degree that the actual seed should be digested. Hence on the one hand the growth of that soft, sweet, pulpy casing which we call fruit; and on the other hand the frequent enclosing of the actual seed in a hard or unsavoury shell, and the secretion within it of essences which are destructive to animal life: paralleled, *pari passu*, in the animal world by the collateral development of a nervous structure at the entrance of the alimentary canal which is pleasurably affected by the one, while it is painfully affected by the other, and of a general structure on which the former produce beneficial effects and the latter injurious ones.*

Finally, we pass on to the third region of the mouth, whose sensations are in direct sympathy with the stomach. This is the lower part of the tongue and threshold of the pharynx. Like the last portion examined it is supplied with

* At what point in the vertebrate series this special gustatory affection begins, and how far it is similar in all species with regard to what are relatively to us sweet and bitter substances, are very difficult questions to decide in the absence of subjective information, which is here in the present state of science the most important evidence obtainable. It may be doubted, too, how far it undergoes modification in the carnivora, and even in the ruminants, to meet the special circumstances of their food. Probably sweet and bitter substances affect birds much as they do us; and the majority of the mammalia show a liking for sugar and a distaste for bitter substances: but I have only gone back to the Quadrumana in the text, because it is with them that the habits of feeding first approximate sufficiently to our own to justify an argument from heredity.

twigs of the glosso-pharyngeal, but the difference of sensation and of irritant imply a difference in the fibres and their central organs. It is here that we discriminate that class of feelings which Professor Bain terms Relishes and Disgusts. These yield us pleasures and pains more closely connected with the necessary vital functions than any others of the gustatory sense, because they are almost purely premonitory of the action of the stomach upon the food swallowed. Consequently, they vary much with the state of the appetite and the digestive apparatus. Roast and boiled meats, rich vegetables and roots, made dishes, butter and oils, oysters or crabs, and similar food stuffs, arouse sensations of this class. When they affect the sense favourably, the feeling is a peculiarly sensuous one, hard to describe but familiar to all, which urges us to push the morsel further and further down the mouth. This action is a sort of semi-voluntary anticipation of the peristaltic contractions, and its occurrence is a probable indication that the digestive organs will not be injuriously affected, as there is great continuity of structure and innervation between the lower part of the mouth and the portion of the stomach adjoining it. The pleasure is doubtless referable to the renewed normal stimulation of the nerves, succeeding a period of intermission and repair, as it passes away after eating sufficiently, and gives place to a feeling of satiety, and a repugnance to any further stimulation. On the other hand, when the morsel is one which will not probably prove digestible in the momentary state of the organs, it gives rise to a peculiar discomfort, known as a Disgust. This is not exactly a pain, nor does it arise, apparently, from any directly disintegrative action. Probably it is rather an anticipatory symptom of that violent retching whereby the stomach ultimately rejects indigestible and offensive matters. Thus some people have great physical difficulty in swallowing cod-liver oil or putrid meat; by others they are swallowed, but soon rejected; while a few persons cannot control the automatic act of expulsion as soon as they reach the lower part of the tongue. Similar confirmation is yielded by the disgust for food which we experience during sea-sickness or other derangement of the stomach. In short, the whole province of this region is to pronounce finally upon the digestibility of food which has passed the tactual examination at the lips and the tip of the tongue, as well as the gustatory ordeal of the middle region. While the tactual fibres reject whatever will prove destructive to the tissues generally, and the pure gustatory district refuses whatever will produce special pathological effects upon the internal organs, the lower portion of the oral cavity decides the minor question whether the food offered it will prove digestible or will be a cause of violent expulsory effort to the muscles of digestion. All this, however, must be accepted only of the healthy natural appetite and digestion of primitive man; as, in our present state, we often find comparatively simple meats, which yielded us no disgust, prove difficult to digest. The popular belief that our likes and dislikes are the best guide to what is desirable for us is founded upon a truth of our original nature, though much obscured by our present artificial life: for as a rule whatever is relished will prove wholesome, and whatever rouses disgust will prove nauseating. It is only because in civilized cookery we mix together so many contrary tastes, and disguise the natural flavour of food, thereby vitiating our palates and overworking our digestive organs, that this simple truth is so often called in question.

Before we pass away from the sense of Taste, it will be as well to mention a few of its peculiarities which bear upon Æsthetic Feeling. Properly speaking no sensation of Taste can be classed as æsthetic; but there are differences between them in this respect, some approaching more nearly to the æsthetic level and others receding very far from it. Feelings belonging to the class last examined, relishes and disgusts, are so closely connected with life-serving function as to be very widely removed from the standard of Æsthetics. We associate no idea of the sort with roast goose, mince pies, pâté-de-foie-gras, or buttered toast. On the other hand there is a faint approach to the æsthetic level in tastes of the pure gustatory class, the sweets and the bitters. Sugar and honey, peaches and melons, wormwood and aloes, do not carry with them the same idea of grossness and bodily functions as the previous instances. Consequently, while the first, even in their ideal form, are almost impossible in Art, either pictorial or poetical, the latter, when idealized and surrounded by other æsthetic objects, form considerable elements for the painter and versifier. Pictures containing such factors as fruit, honey-comb, filberts, or red wines are common with both; but they scarcely venture to introduce beef, bacon, beer, or gin.* Of course, in every case, great

* Certain pictures of the Dutch School which do so can scarcely be reckoned as adverse instances. Though their admirable execution may command our praise, their subject must be regarded as outside the æsthetic class.

allowance must be made for complication with the æsthetic element of sight, and sundry emotional factors in the total effect; yet I think we may safely say that part of the difference lies in the sense of Taste itself. Flavours of this higher sort are distinguished in ordinary language as *delicate;* a word which at once implies æsthetic descriminativeness. Soft and smooth substances like jellies produce a similar impression. In short, those objects which rouse tastes or disgusts strongly in sympathy with the stomach are very far removed from the æsthetic class; those more remotely connected with digestion approach that class at a less distance. This point will, however, receive further attention at a later stage, and is only introduced here by anticipation lest the reader should fail to see what connexion exists between the present analysis of the lower senses and the general question of Æsthetics.

§ 3. *Smell.*

After our lengthy treatment of Taste it will not be necessary to enter quite so fully into the kindred sense of Smell.

The organ of smell is situated within the nasal cavity. It possesses, like the tongue, a mucous membrane copiously supplied with nervous fibres, terminating in special bodies, analogous in function with the tactile corpuscles and lingual papillæ, which are known as olfactory cells. The gaseous bodies which reach the olfactory chamber act directly upon these cells. But just as bodies must be in solution to affect the tongue, so they must be volatilized to affect the nose.

The nose may be divided into two sensitive regions. The first, situated at the entrance of the nasal cavity, is supplied with nerves of touch from the trigeminus, and yields sensations which are mainly tactual. The second, situated in the olfactory chamber, is supplied, in addition to these, with the pure olfactory nerve, and yields sensations of its own peculiar character, most of which are in sympathy with the stomach and the organ of taste.

The object of Smell is two-fold, and this makes its treatment a little more complicated than that of Taste. In the first place it is an anticipatory Taste, and guides us towards those objects which are useful for food, while it strongly repels us from those which will prove injurious. In the second place it is premonitory of the effect upon the lungs of the gases inhaled, being gratified by those of a pure and healthy nature, while it is irritated by such as will prove prejudicial to the blood or pulmonary tissues. We shall have to consider its various phenomena in both these lights.

The tactual sensibility of the nose is due to its trigeminal fibres and is excited by those volatile bodies which possess the power of chemically stimulating the nerves of touch in other situations. Ammonia, which as we have seen acts powerfully on the skin and the tongue, is a pungent stimulant to the nose. So are pepper, mustard, cayenne, and the other bodies of that class. Acetic acid and similar very sour substances, if capable of volatilization, affect the nose in a certain distinctive manner, which bears some analogy to their lingual effect. Alcohols and many ethers also produce a slight stinging sensation. In every one of these cases the likeness to the instance of Taste is very striking. An extremely small quantity of the irritant is agreeable as stimulation, but only to the dulled and blunted nervous centres of adults: while even with them a slight excess brings on the painful and destructive degree of action. Furthermore, each of these stimulants, when inhaled in large quantities, exercises a destructive action upon the tissues of the lungs; while, if swallowed in excess, they will prove injurious, as we have already seen, to the coats of the stomach and intestines. So that we have here a double instance of the establishment of an organic consensus, the pungency at once warning us off from inhaling the irritant vapour in any large amount, and deterring us from making any further experiment by putting the body whence the vapour arises into our mouths. Children and dogs are generally sufficiently instructed by the nose not to eat anything on which mustard or pepper has been spread: and the violent irritation caused by large volumes of pungent vapour soon urges us to remove the smelling bottle, or to rush from the loaded atmosphere into the open air, as the case may be.

Passing on to the pure olfactory sensibility, we shall find it convenient to take separately the two classes of sensations which yield indications of the probable effects upon the stomach and the lungs respectively of bodies which give rise to smell. In the first of these two classes we notice that the scent of cooked meats and other relishes is pleasing so long as we are hungry, but becomes distasteful as soon as we have eaten to repletion. This shows a sympathy with the stomach exactly analogous to that of Taste. Similarly, the fragrance of peaches, oranges, pine-apples, strawberries, and other fruits is pleasurable, and strongly suggests the flavour, thus acting as an incentive towards eating them. So, too, with wines, coffee, and aromatic drinks. On the other hand, the smell of decaying animal matter is very offensive, and acts as a strong deterrent against any attempt to taste it. Dead bodies cause us to avoid their neighbourhood; and the smell of boiling tallow, in a putrescent state, as in the manufacture of soap, is sufficient to drive us to a distance immediately. Putrid cheese or butter, bad fish, high meat, are always unpleasant to the unsophisticated sense. Decaying vegetables, though not quite so disagreeable, rouse a recognizable feeling of disgust. Those which contain large quantities of sulphur yield nauseating stenches. Nothing is simpler than to suppose that the pleasing class of smells stimulate the nerves in the normal manner; as to the unpleasant ones, I would venture to suggest as a possible explanation that they may set up at once a faint disintegrative action analogous to that set up in wounds by putrescent germs, as in hospital gangrene. It is hardly necessary to add that such an arrangement is what we should naturally expect from the consensus of the organs, as the pleasantly-scented objects of this kind are mainly those which are desirable as food, and the unpleasant ones those which, if swallowed, would produce nausea or other morbid action. Moreover, as the organs of Taste and Smell are continuous in their lower portions, the sympathy with the stomach is readily understood.

In the second class of odours, those in sympathy with the

lungs, we see that fresh air, and the pure, innocuous perfumes of flowers and fruits are pleasant; while foul air, overloaded with carbonic acid and decaying animal matter in minute particles, is unpleasant. This form of discomfort, however, has its seat rather in the lungs themselves than in the respiratory canal, and its opposite is the gratification resulting from a gulp of pure air, and the consequent renewal of healthy pulmonary action. More strictly olfactory is the unpleasant odour of the poisonous gases, such as sulphuretted, phosphuretted, and arseniuretted hydrogen, or bisulphide of carbon. Why the nose should be unfavourably impressed by these is, teleologically speaking, obvious: while the fact that these gases rapidly destroy organic tissues enables us to bring their case at once under our general law of pain. The opposite instances are found in the perfumes of flowers, which, though not so easily explicable, may be considered as owing their agreeable nature to the mere fact of due stimulation within the normal limits. Smell being with us a mere relic (as is shown by the shrivelled dimensions of the central organs which represent the olfactory lobes of lower animals), we may probably trace back these pleasures to the scents of fruits and flowers, which are evidently given them, like their colour and sweetness, as allurements for insects, birds, and mammals, to promote cross-fertilization and the dissemination of seeds. Hence we may regard them as forming another instance of that consensus between fauna and flora which we noticed in the case of Taste.* The agreeable scents will thus be

* It may be added that the pleasure felt by coarse nervous organizations in

analogous to the sweet tastes; a view which is borne out by the fact that when very largely increased in intensity or duration, as in jasmine or stephanotis, they merely result in an excessive cloying, like that of honey in the gustatory sense. This unpleasant feeling is simply one of over-stimulation; it differs widely from the actively disagreeable and presumably destructive action of the poisonous gases.

If it be objected that some poisonous gases, such as carbonic oxide, do not smell disagreeable, the answer must be that this is one of those failures of adaptation—those incomplete establishments of the consensus, which must always be expected in all imperfect organisms. Just as the tongue does not always discriminate poisonous solids and liquids, so the nose does not always discriminate poisonous gases. Yet even here we may notice two qualifying circumstances. In the first place, though carbonic oxide is poisonous, it does not, like the strongly-scented gaseous poisons, act rapidly upon organic tissues; so that it is analogous to those insipid substances which have not sufficient chemical activity to affect the gustatory nerves. In the second place, it is not a gas which is likely to occur in the environment of uncivilized man or his ancestors; while the gases formed by the decomposition of animal matters, absence of drainage, miasmatic effluvia of tropical swamps, and similar causes, are constantly to be found in such circumstances; and of course the organism can only be expected to adapt itself to those agencies in the environment which

the perfume of musk has been considered by some as a remnant of the gratification derived by lower animals from sexual odours.

most frequently and directly affect it. So that we need never concern ourselves in this inquiry with those sapid or odorous bodies which are mere laboratory products, but only with those which occur spontaneously in nature.

In estimating the place of Smell in the æsthetic hierarchy of the senses, we are led to notice one striking peculiarity which lends it a special interest in connexion with our present subject. Of all the senses of man, Smell is the one which is least intellectual and most purely emotional. We may occasionally employ it to discriminate the contents of a bottle or the nature of a doubtful substance; but for the most part it yields us relatively large emotional waves, and relatively small intellectual information. This is not the case in the lower animals. The carnivora use it to track their prey; the ruminants to escape their enemies. Hence, in them it is connected with a fully-developed central organ. But in man the olfactory sensibility is a mere relic, which has outlived its principal uses. Accordingly, its central organ has dwindled away, and it has come to be almost purely a source of pleasure and pain. This peculiarity helps to raise it almost to the æsthetic level. It is true that those odours which have obvious reference to vital organic processes (such as the smell of roast meats and fish, on the one hand, or of decaying animal matter on the other) have no pretence of reaching the æsthetic standard of disinterestedness. Accordingly the pleasant odours of this class are inadmissible into Poetry, even in the ideal form; while the unpleasant ones, commonly known by the disagreeable name of stinks, are so loathsome as to form the ne plus ultra of the æsthetically hideous. But the fragrance of fruits and spices very nearly approaches the requisite freedom from life-serving function; because the taste which it suggests is of the kind least intimately connected with organic wants. And when we pass on from these lower instances to those sweet odours which are utterly unconnected with the organs of digestion, such as the perfume of a rose, a violet, or a lily-of-the-valley, the smell of new-mown hay, the aroma of newly-ploughed land, we feel that these, even in the actuality, are in almost every respect raised into the æsthetic class. Moreover, the perfume-exciting qualities of the rose or the violet are not destroyed in the act of smelling them, as the taste-exciting qualities of a peach or a pear are destroyed in the act of eating them. So that we have here, to a considerable extent, that absence of monopoly which we saw to be one of the distinguishing marks of æsthetic objects. And if these objects in the actuality arouse feelings so nearly approaching the æsthetic level, we naturally find their ideal representation entering largely into the composition of Poetry. Of course here, too, we must make great allowances for beauty of form and colour, but we cannot doubt that some part in the poetical effectiveness of fragrant flowers must be attributed to the sense of Smell.

§ 4. *Cookery and Perfumery.*

There are two arts which, though not æsthetic, stand in the same relation to the senses of Taste and Smell as painting and music do to those of sight and hearing. Consequently, they throw a little light upon the purely æsthetic arts, and so deserve a few words in passing. Though the pleasures of Taste may occur in connexion with food in its raw state, and though the object of cooking in its simplest form is rather to render food digestible than to make it more palatable, yet in its highest developments the practice of cookery, including therein the whole preparation of food for the table, and the due arrangement of courses, almost rises to the dignity of a fine art, possessing its professors and its cognoscenti.* We saw in the last chapter that the ultimate principle of Æsthetics was the maximum of stimulation with the minimum of fatigue in processes not directly connected with necessary vital functions. Now the rule of cookery is just the same, in those processes which relate to the ingestion of food and drink. The object of a good chef is to lay upon the table a dinner, every dish in which shall stimulate the nerves of taste in different manners, without ever palling or flagging; to alternate and co-ordinate courses so that they shall succeed one another in the most acceptable order, the lighter viands preceding the heavier, and no course spoiling the palate for the succeeding one; and to ensure much variety without any sense of repletion. He prefers clear soups to thick broth, which would too rapidly exhaust the appetite; he carefully assorts the sauces for his fish, adding flavour to cod by oysters, and tempering the richness of whitebait with lemon; he dresses his entrées in the lightest, daintiest, and most piquant style; he cooks his

* Those who wish to see cookery treated au grand sérieux as a fine art, may turn to Brillat-Savarin's *Physiologie du Goût,* or to an amusing brochure on *the Art of Dining,* attributed to Mr. A. Hayward.

joints to a turn; and when the digestive organs are satiated with these more solid viands, he stimulates the taste with game, follows it up with light and delicate pastry, and concludes with fruits, sweetmeats, and ices. He adds olives to clear the palate for the wine, which has also been carefully adapted to each stage of the dinner; hock with the fish, champagne with the joints, and the heavier vintages, such as port, sherry, and Madeira, to finish the repast. Finally, he serves up a cup of full-flavoured coffee, whose delicate yet powerful aroma can still urge on the appetite, when coarser flavours would disgust and weaker ones fail to attract. And yet, if he has been successful, he leaves the digestion unimpaired and the mental powers clear. Every exertion has been made to give the maximum of stimulation with the minimum of fatigue, alike to the organ of taste and to the digestive apparatus. The analogy to the æsthetic arts is obvious; but what gives the sense of purity in the one and of comparative grossness in the other is the presence or absence respectively of ulterior life-serving purposes, besides the fact that food is above all other enjoyments necessarily a matter of strict monopoly.

Perfumery has not been carried to nearly so high a pitch as cookery, and for an obvious reason. Whereas cookery is useful in the preparation of food and only endeavours incidentally to give immediate pleasure, perfumery is not necessarily connected with any life-serving function on the one hand, while on the other it is not susceptible of any high artistic and intellectual combinations. One of our great humorists[1] has indeed given a whimsical account of an imaginary instrument for yielding æsthetic combinations of odours, by means of stoppers opened and shut in certain orders, so as to give rise to harmonies and contrasts, the perfumes being made to succeed one another rapidly by means of a current of air, over which the nose of the amateur was held. But, apart from the mechanical difficulties of such an instrument, there is a fatal physiological objection in the persistence and sameness of the sense of smell, which would prevent that rapid and distinct succession of impressions in time or space which makes possible the delicate harmonies and contrasts of sounds and colours. Hence perfumery has never given rise to an art of any pretension. Moreover, artificial essences never yield the same pure and delicious fragrance as natural flowers and fruits. There is always a sickly tinge about their sweetness. This inability to compete with nature is a fatal objection to perfumery as the basis of a fine art. It is characteristic of the true æsthetic arts generally that they are *more* beautiful than nature, because they gather together all that is lovely, and omit all that is low, discordant or ugly. Thus the Discobolus or the Medici Venus is more beautiful than any living nude human figure, because it combines all the best points of many; a landscape painting is lovelier than reality, because it excludes all unpleasant accompaniments; a great poem takes us into a region of ideal delights; a grand oratorio immeasurably surpasses any natural collection of sounds. But a lily-of-the-valley or a heliotrope is worth all the mille-fleurs or frangipanni that was ever manufactured.

And now, with the light that has been cast upon the pleasures and pains of the lower senses in the present analysis, we may proceed to those higher senses whose pleasures and pains form the chief basis for the purely æsthetic arts of Music, Sculpture, Painting, Architecture, and Poetry.

CHAPTER V.

TOUCH.

§ 1. *Emotional Phenomena of Touch.*

VERY little need be said about the tactual sense, and yet that little is well entitled to the dignity of a separate chapter. The science of Æsthetics is but slightly concerned with Touch, because it forms the exact antipodes of smell, in being almost purely intellectual and very little emotional. For this there are two reasons. Touch proper, being only affected by pressures, cannot yield us appreciable pains; since, when the painful stage is reached, we refer the crushing or laceration to the general organic sensibility. Again, the skin being in almost constant contact with surrounding objects, the sense of Touch does not need special stimulation, as its organs seldom or never have long intervals of repair; and so it cannot yield us any acute pleasures. Nevertheless, on the other hand, Touch is the first of the senses, in the order of examination which we have adopted, to afford us feelings which may be unreservedly classed as æsthetic, in the actuality as well as in the idea. Tastes and Smells may become subjects of art in the representation alone, but Touch enters into its composition directly. We will therefore run rapidly over the few emotional feelings which are yielded by this sense.

Rough substances, like flannel or horse-hair, placed next the skin, chafe it and give rise to painful feelings. Soft and smooth ones, on the contrary, such as silk and fine linen, only arouse the normal amount of nervous action, and are accordingly agreeable, or at least neutral. A faint voluptuous feeling is experienced for the first few moments after putting on silk underclothing. A fly, a hair, or a drop of moisture, affecting any thin-skinned part (for example, the neck or cheeks) causes an excessive stimulation which, though not exactly painful, is extremely annoying. The palm of the hand, being unusually well supplied with tactile corpuscles, affords us some more special emotional effects. There is a peculiar discomfort in running one's hand over a rough or gritty surface, owing partly to the faint tendency to abrasion, partly to the constant impeding of motion and consequent twitching or retraction, which of course implies wasteful expenditure of energy. On moving the finger tips over a piece of velvet wall-paper, such as is often used in dining-rooms, we are conscious of a jarring sensation, analogous to that aroused in the auditory sense by the grating of a pencil on a slate, and doubtless due to the excessive, jerky, and wasteful stimulation of the tactile corpuscles. The gritty coloured papers sold for decorating dishes set the teeth on edge when touched: so do brick and emery cloth. There is a corresponding gratification in the easy and unimpeded gliding of the fingers over a perfectly smooth surface. Hence a portion of the pleasure with which we regard polish on stone or marble, glass or porcelain, varnish on furniture, and soft fabrics like silk or velvet, is doubtless due to tactual feelings, real or ideal; though allowances must be made for the visual gratifications of lustre and the flowing form. Indeed glossiness, though doubtless agreeable in itself to the sense of sight, is mainly prized as the visual symbol of tactual smoothness. Rough-sawn marble sends through us the peculiar discordant jar produced by jerky stimulation, which will be more fully explained in the chapter on Hearing: when polished, it yields us a pleasant sense of harmonious and regular excitation. A simple confirmatory experiment can be tried by passing the hand first over the under surface of a mantelpiece (which is usually left in the rough state) and then over the polished top. The most sensuous variety of this pleasure is found in stroking a seal-skin, a cat's back, or a piece of satin. Softness here complicates the effect; smoothness alone gives pleasurable qualities to a mahogany table, a tortoise-shell card-case, or a rose-wood desk. The handles of instruments, being often grasped, ought to be specially smooth: hence those used at table or in the toilet (as well as the keys of pianos) are usually fitted with bone, ivory, or mother-of-pearl; commoner tools have them of polished hard-wood. Door-handles and the knobs of house-bells are made of porcelain or smooth metal. Rough iron is very disagreeable to grasp; the tongs and the poker are as bright as silver. In an æsthetically-furnished room, leaving out of consideration for the present the visual elements, part of the effect is due to the smoothness of the walnut sofas and tables, the soft satin or tabouret coverings, and the morocco easy-chairs; and part to the suggestion of ease and comfort in their luxurious stuffing, and their contour adapted to the natural positions of the limbs. Even in food, the pleasantness of jellies, custards, creams, and ices, is partly owing to their softness and the absence of any necessity for muscular effort in masticating or swallowing them. Strawberries and peaches melt in the mouth. On the other hand, grittiness in food is disagreeable and often painful, while toughness gives unnecessary work to the jaws. Throughout, whatever compels or suggests excessive effort, waste of energy, or abrasion of skin is unpleasant and ugly: whatever is clearly free from these defects is pleasant and beautiful.

§ 2. *Æsthetic Value of Touch.*

Of course the examples cited above of pleasures and pains connected with the sense of Touch do not all equally come under the æsthetic class. Those which relate to food and to underclothing are clearly too closely allied to essential vital functions. Softness, again, is inextricably bound up with the sexual instinct. But the purely disinterested pleasures and pains of smoothness and roughness belong entirely to the æsthetic group. They possess all the characteristics which were enumerated above in the chapter on the Differentia of Æsthetics. They are very remotely or not at all connected with necessary life-serving function. The pleasurable ones amongst them are marked by the fact that they arouse the maximum of stimulation in the organs affected, with the minimum of fatigue or waste; while the disagreeable ones are marked merely by their failure to comply with this requirement, not by any active or violent destruction of tissue. Their objects are not monopolized, nor are they destroyed in the act of enjoyment. And, finally, their elements are so slightly pleasurable or painful, as the case may be, that they are scarcely emotionally cognized, but rather intellectually discriminated. While sweets and bitters, perfumes and stenches, yield comparatively large and recognizable waves of pleasure and pain, smooth or rough objects yield feelings whose emotional character is only recognized upon mature deliberation. They almost escape us in ordinary life, and only rise into importance when they are so combined with many others (such as those of form and colour) as to arouse a complex thrill of beauty or ugliness. Indeed, a great part of the displeasure felt at rough or rugged objects is due to the impression of bad workmanship; and a great part of the gratification aroused by smooth and polished objects is due to the consciousness of finish and workmanlike or artistic care. We find, as before observed, that the components of the æsthetic thrill are very faint emotional waves, but that by many re-inforcements they become at last sufficiently voluminous for conscious recognition.

Accordingly, elements derived from the sense of Touch enter freely into the various arts, both in the actuality and in the idea. The earliest stone implements are rough and angular; but some belonging to the neo-lithic and modern periods have attained a polish and smoothness which would not disgrace the most civilized lapidary. Savages love to polish cocoa-nuts and other hard seeds, as well as clubs and precious stones. The Egyptians made their granite figures as smooth as glass. In their fully developed forms, the arts still plentifully employ tactual factors. In Music, it is clearly impossible that they can take any part; but we find them widely employed in Painting, Sculpture, Architecture, and (ideally) in Poetry; while they are almost supreme in decorative art. It will only be necessary to mention in detail the coating or varnish upon oil pictures, the smoothness of their surface, and the inartistic effect of blotches which rise distinctly above the general level: while ideal softness of silks, furs, wool, and foliage, and, above all, of human flesh, is a common pictorial device. Marble statuettes gain by polish, and bronze has the tactual element strongly developed. Granite or syenite pedestals point in the same direction. We almost instinctively test a polished pillar with the hand. But it is in Architecture, and more especially in internal decoration, that the tactual sense becomes most important. Mosaics, intaglio work, encaustic pavements, malachite and porphyry vases, all owe much to it. Precious stones, jet, and amber take a high polish. Rough earthenware is varnished over; and porcelain or majolica have an external coat of glazing which hides their gritty surfaces. The tomb of Napoléon at the Invalides, with all its gewgaw surroundings, yet impresses us by its manual elaboration. Japanese lacquer, buhl cabinets, marble or ivory decorations, at once inform us by their lustre or glossiness of their smooth texture. In fact almost all art-furniture (as opposed to mere upholstery,) derives a large part of its æsthetic character from tactual elements. So also do the richer kinds of dress,—silk, satin, velvet, cashmere, broadcloth, furs, swansdown, grebe, ostrich feathers, lace, and kid. Ermine and sealskin deserve special mention. In all, great allowances must be made for the emotional element of costliness. Finally, every one of these objects which is beautiful in the actuality, becomes in the idea a possible component of Poetry. But here again we trench upon the ground of later chapters, as is almost inevitable when dealing with a subject so full of complications and re-involutions as Æsthetic Feeling.

Beside these consciously-sought artistic pleasures, certain æsthetic objects occur spontaneously in nature which owe part of their beauty to the tactual sense. Grassy slopes suggest the notion of an easy couch, as do also mossy or fern-clad banks. Ice has a glassy surface, and freshly fallen snow, in spite of its coldness, besides impressing us visually by its purity and sparkle, spreads a coat of yielding softness over the hard roads and rugged hillside. Poets accordingly dwell chiefly on the fleeciness of its gently falling flakes. Chrysanthemums, dahlias, and immortelles owe part of their ungraceful effect to the stiffness of their petals: roses, violets, and anemones, on the contrary, please us by their agreeable softness. Rose petals are the poetical embodiment of delicacy, and the school-book story of the Sybarite has given them the stamp of conventional illustration. To "die of a rose in aromatic pain" is our idea of æsthetic fastidiousness. Those odious parodies of artistic products, wax and paper flowers, are indebted to their stiff materials for part of their hideous vulgarity; though I believe their main failing to be that, like artificial perfumes, they fall far short of nature, instead of surpassing it.

To sum up, we see that Touch is very little an emotional sense, and consequently very little an æsthetic one; but that out of the few emotional feelings which it yields, a considerable proportion belong to the strictly æsthetic class, and that it is accordingly entitled to rank with sight and hearing as forming part of the basis for the fine arts and for Poetry.

CHAPTER VI.

HEARING.

§ 1. *Characteristics of the Higher Senses.*

THOUGH we saw in the last chapter that Touch must be allowed a place in the immediately æsthetic class, yet the two higher senses of Sight and Hearing deserve to occupy a pedestal of their own which raises them far above those hitherto examined. The main ground for this distinction may be gathered from the following considerations.

The nerves of Taste and Smell are not individually discriminative: that is, each one of them does not yield us a different sensation. For the most part, large masses of gustatory and olfactory nerves are stimulated at once; and their connected centres afford us identical factors of consciousness. But every single fibre of the optic and auditory nerves seems capable of differential stimulation, and yields us a distinct and separate impression. Hence, while stimulation and fatigue usually extend over large tracts of the olfactory and gustatory systems, every single fibre of the optic and auditory apparatus, with its connected centre, is probably capable of separate pleasure and separate fatigue.

Again, while the lower senses are exposed to directly disintegrative and violently painful action, or to strong pleasurable excitement, the nerves of the two higher and specially æsthetic senses are so delicate in calibre, and so carefully guarded from surrounding agencies that they generally undergo only comparatively slight stimulations from their proper excitants; so that their pains are for the most part merely those of fatigue rather than of violent disintegration, and their pleasures those of delicate and harmonious action rather than of powerful and long-intermitted stimulation. The optic and auditory nerves are not liable to be scratched, burned, bruised, or attacked by chemical agents, but only to be wearied by over use or jarred by discordant sounds and colours.

Furthermore, as these senses influence our conduct mainly through the intellect, they are not liable to pleasures and pains of the directly anticipatory sort. Desirable food-stuffs do not gratify the eye or ear, nor do disagreeable ones disintegrate them excessively.* Hence they are little connected directly with life-serving functions; and their pleasures are mainly those of such due stimulation as will keep up their normal efficiency; while their pains are those of such overwork as will render the structures less useful in future.†

* The influence of bright-coloured fruits, berries, and flowers on the growth of Æsthetic Feelings will be discussed in the chapter on Sight.

† Even here, however, we find some approach to the establishment of that consensus which is the automatic protection of the organism. The instinctive dread of the serpentine form which pervades the whole of humanity has been ingeniously referred to a hereditary terror, ingrained in the nervous constitution, surviving from a period when our early ancestors were specially exposed to the attacks of poisonous snakes as their chief enemies. The hatred of cows for dogs (prior to all experience on either side) is probably a reminiscence

But the most important distinction of all is that which holds between the rates of exhaustion and repair in the higher and lower senses respectively. Tastes and smells can be endured at a considerable height of stimulation for a considerable period of time; and when the stimulant is withdrawn, the sensation persists for a few seconds. But after fatigue at length sets in, a long interval of reparation is necessary before the structures recover their excitability. The organs of Sight and Hearing, on the contrary, are easily exhausted and quickly repaired. A glance at the sun dazzles our eyes, and we see a negative image accordingly wherever we look. The boom of a cannon deafens our ears, and we cannot for a few seconds hear any lesser sounds. Even the infinitesimally rapid flash of an electric spark is sufficient to weary the delicate nerves of sight. But, except in such extreme cases, the eye and the ear are quickly repaired after each stimulation. There is reason to believe that the optic fibres and terminal organs are repaired, in ordinary cases, seventeen times per second, and those of the auditory nerves thirty-three times per second. To this peculiarity we must in part attribute their great power of intellectual discrimination; for though this is due, so far as regards the variety of possible sensations, to the immense number of fibres which

of the days when their respective ancestors, the aurochs and the wolf, fought one another in the forests of central Europe. Young chickens, which dart automatically at a fly, run cowering to their mother from the sight of a hawk. The roar of carnivores has a startling effect upon almost all other animals; and thunder or loud explosions terrify us instinctively. But these cases only show a nascent consensus, very different from the developed correspondence in the lower senses.

may be differentially stimulated, yet so far as concerns their separateness in time and rapidity of succession, it depends upon the immediate reparatory qualities of the nerves. So that the same properties which make the eye and ear our most discriminative organs, also bestow upon them their æsthetic value. For, owing to the immense variety of their fibres, and the rapidity of their exhaustion and repair, we have constantly induced in their several portions partial fatigues which are very slight in amount, and partial stimulations which excite small areas of their terminal surface, in a comparatively high state of nutrition, and consequently ready to yield pleasurable feelings as soon as stimulated. Accordingly, they, above all others, are subjects for that minute intellectual discrimination which we recognized as one of the marks that differentiate the Æsthetic Feelings from other pleasures and pains.

§ 2. *Air-waves and the Organ for their Perception.**

If we move a fan rapidly through the atmosphere, we are conscious of a blast of air in contact with the face. If a heavy weight falls on the ground in our neighbourhood, the jar is communicated to our bodies. If a cannon is fired close to the spot where we stand, we are strongly shaken by the concussion. In all these cases, masses of air are set in violent motion, impinge upon our bodies, and cause an ordinary sensation of Touch.

* In all the strictly physiological portion of this chapter I owe my acknowledgments to Helmholtz's *Sensations of Tone*, which I have used chiefly in Mr. Ellis's translation.

But besides these larger and easily recognized motions of the air, there are others of a smaller and less discriminable class. When any body, solid, liquid, or gaseous, impinges upon another with any considerable energy, aerial undulations are set up whose presence, though not manifested to our sense of Touch, can easily be made visible by means of very small pendulous bodies, allowed to swing freely. Such bodies will be set in motion by the waves so generated. Of these waves there are two kinds. The first kind results when the body impinged upon immediately returns to a position of rest: the second kind results when the body impinged upon continues to vibrate freely. The waves generated by the first are irregular and indefinite; those generated by the second are perfectly regular and perform a fixed number of vibrations in a unit of time until the bodies generating them have returned to a position of rest. To take specific examples, the first kind of wave is produced when a stone falls on the ground, or when the fist is struck upon the table: the second kind of wave is produced when a tuning fork or a violin string receives a blow, and continues to vibrate freely till the energy it has received is dissipated by friction.

Now the aerial waves thus set in motion, though capable of producing some slight mechanical effects, are too small, for the most part, to affect our nerves of touch. But we have a special nervous end-organ so arranged as to be specially sensitive to these slight waves; and this organ is the ear. It collects the minute undulations, concentrates and strengthens them by a series of ingenious devices, and finally directs them upon the terminals of an important nerve, which conveys the information they afford to the auditory centre, and so at last to the higher co-ordinating regions of the brain.

It will be observed that I have carefully abstained from using the dangerous and misleading word *Sound* with relation to these aerial undulations, because that word really implies a reference to our sense of Hearing; and I think it important to impress upon the reader that these waves do not objectively differ from any others, but are governed by the ordinary mechanical laws of elastic fluids. It is only when cognized through the sense of Hearing that they become distinctively *Sounds;* and many such waves which cannot be so cognized, owing to their very rapid or very slow vibrations, are objectively indistinguishable from sound-waves proper, that is, from those which lie within the limits for producing the auditory sensation. For the present, therefore, we shall only regard the undulations from the strictly objective stand-point, as waves of air.

Let us see, then, with necessary brevity, what is the conformation of this specialised organ by which we become conscious of aerial vibrations. We will only look at such of its parts as are absolutely essential to a proper comprehension of our subject, referring the reader for details to morphological and physiological treatises on the ear.

The outer portion of the human ear consists of an external passage, through which the air-waves are conducted to the tympanum or drum; which is an internal cavity, separated from the passage by a thin circular membrane. Beyond the drum, again, is situated the labyrinth, a cavity filled with fluid, on whose walls are expanded the ends of the fibres belonging to the auditory nerve. The object of the passage is to collect the aerial waves; that of the drum is to conduct them with sufficient force into the fluid of the labyrinth; and that of the last-named portion to excite the nerve-terminations themselves. In these various operations the parts named are assisted by many minor pieces of mechanism which need not here be detailed.

In order to explain the manner in which the aerial undulations are finally converted into nervous stimulation we must look at some analogous phenomena in the outer world. It is a well-known fact of physics that any oscillating body may be set in motion by very slight external energies, provided they are applied with the same periodic recurrences as those of the body's own vibrations. If a pendulum or a church bell receives a number of impulses, each very slight in comparison with the mass to be moved, but so timed that every fresh impulse coincides with the period of the body's swing, it can soon be set in motion in spite of the smallness of the motive power, because each impulse reinforces the last at the exact moment when such reinforcement will produce the greatest effect. Conversely, such a body once set in motion can be easily brought to rest by a number of comparatively slight checks given it in the course of its vibration. Now we find outside the human or animal organism that certain elastic bodies, such as tuning-forks, violin-strings, and stretched membranes, possess a natural period of vibration, and that when the aerial undulations produced by another body in motion impinge upon them, they produce a sympathetic vibration, provided their recurring periods coincide exactly (or, in some cases, approximately) with the natural periods of the body sympathetically excited. Without entering for the present into special details, it will be sufficient here to remark that among the elastic bodies in which sympathetic vibrations can thus be excited may probably be classed the nerve-terminations of the human ear. Their terminal expansions are connected with certain small elastic appendages; and there is every reason to believe that each of these appendages possesses a natural period of its own, and can consequently be set in sympathetic vibration by such aerial waves as exactly or nearly coincide with its own period.* Moreover, each of them is connected with its corresponding fibres by a mechanism which is apparently adapted to communicate to the fibre the excitement which the appendage has received. Finally, a differential mode of sensation seems to be attached to the central termination of each fibre, so that the total sensation received depends upon the various fibres differentially affected and their combinations. Such is, in its roughest form, the modern theory of Hearing. We must now expand it slightly by enquiring what are the various modes of stimulation thus differentially cognized, and what their subjective counterparts.

* In the auditory apparatus of certain small crabs, Hensen observed different particular hairs in sympathetic vibration with air-waves of different particular frequencies.

§ 3. *Varieties of Air-waves and their Equivalents in Consciousness.*

We have seen that air-waves, originally set in motion by the impact of one body upon another, impinge upon the ear, through the mechanism of the tympanum and the labyrinth, set up sympathetic vibrations in the elastic bodies which are attached to the terminals of the nerves, and thus communicate a stimulation to the fibres themselves. The impulse so imparted to the auditory centre is there subjectively cognized as *Sound.* We have next to enquire what are the various modes of aerial undulation, and what the corresponding varieties of Sounds.

The first great distinction between air-waves is the one already drawn of those which are produced by a single impact and those which are produced by the continuous vibration of an elastic body. The latter are periodic and regular, the former non-periodic and irregular. But if the ear is to be differentially excited by these different stimulants, and so to cognize them separately, it must have special organs for the perception of each; and the appendages of these special organs must be set in sympathetic motion by one or the other kind of stimulant respectively. Now we find in external nature that some bodies are readily set in motion by irregular and non-periodic waves, but that such bodies only continue in motion for comparatively short periods, instead of vibrating freely for a considerable time: while on the other hand certain other elastic bodies are not set in motion by non-periodic waves, but only answer to undulations whose periods exactly or very closely coincide with their own, in which case a sympathetic vibration is set up and augmented by the recurring impacts of the air-waves. In the labyrinth of the ear we find sets of nervous structures which apparently answer to each of these conditions. In its outer portion, known as the vestibule, and in certain of its windings called the ampullæ, are nervous terminations whose construction leads us to suppose that they are readily excited in sympathy with irregular agitations of short duration: and the sensations aroused in connection with these stimulations are cognized in the auditory centre as *Noises.* The deepest recess of the labyrinth consists of a snail-shaped cavity known as the cochlea, on whose walls are arranged an immense number of small bodies, called after their discoverer Corti's organs, each of which, apparently, is capable of sympathetic vibration only under the influence of a regular undulation whose periodic recurrences closely coincide with its own natural period. These bodies are connected with separate fibres, and when the stimulations thus received are communicated to the brain they are cognized as *Musical Tones.*

Again, air-waves of either class may differ in size, or, as it is oftener expressed, in amplitude of oscillation; that is to say, in distance from crest to crest. Upon this objective difference in the waves depends the subjective difference of *Loudness* and its opposite. When the waves are very great in size, the resulting sound is said to be very loud: as the size diminishes, the sound becomes less and less. In short, loudness is the subjective concomitant of intensity in stimulation. It does not depend upon the particular fibres excited, but upon the amount of the excitation. When we pull aside a violin-string and then allow it to vibrate freely, its excursions are at first considerable, during which period the sound is loud; as it parts slowly with its energy, the excursions gradually decrease, and the sound lessens till it dies away.

Next, let us confine our attention to the second class of air-waves, those which, proceeding from a regularly oscillating body, perform equal numbers of vibrations in equal times, and give rise to Musical Tones. It is clear that these may differ greatly in the number of vibrations which they execute in a given unit of time,—say, for example, a second. Every body capable of producing such undulations has a certain fixed number of its own, which under similar circumstances it always yields. This number may be altered by some alteration in the circumstances of the body (for example, in a string, by lengthening or shortening it; in a finger-glass, by increasing or lessening the quantity of water), but when all other circumstances remain the same, the number of vibrations per second is constant. Fortunately we possess an instrument, the siren, by means of which we can produce undulations of any desired frequency per second. It consists, in principle, of an air-box with an immovable cover, pierced by a fixed number of holes; on top of which is a movable metal disk, similarly pierced, the holes being arranged at such an angle that the disk can be driven round by a blast from a bellows. Each time that the upper and under holes coincide, a puff of air escapes, and we can reckon the number of escapes, or, in other words, the number of waves generated, by means of a dial attached. In conjunction with this instrument we may use certain bottle-shaped resonators, over one of whose open ends is stretched an elastic membrane, against which a drop of sealing-wax is suspended by a delicate thread.* Now we find that when we so adjust the siren as to produce undulations which recur with a certain given frequency per second, the membrane of the resonator begins to vibrate sympathetically, and the little pendulum of sealing-wax is violently agitated. But only waves of that particular frequency will produce this result: to all others the membrane is perfectly passive.† We may arrange a series of these resonators in such an order that as the number of undulations per second produced by the siren is increased, one after another of the membranes is sympathetically set in motion. Now, in the human ear, Helmholtz has shown with great probability that Corti's organs in the cochlea, or snail-shaped cavity of the labyrinth, are a series of elastic bodies, each with a different natural period, arranged in a similar order, so as to be severally excited by recurring undulations having different periods of vibration. Each of

* I prefer this diagrammatic illustration by means of the *acoustic pendulum* to the historical one of Helmholtz's *resonance globes*, because the latter require the use of the auditory nerve, while I am anxious to treat the matter from the objective stand-point alone. Kœnig's mode of demonstration by *manometric flames* would equally well suit my purpose, but it would demand a lengthy and otherwise irrelevant explanation. I am not aware that a series of acoustic pendula, tuned as a gamut of resonators, has ever actually been constructed, but there is nothing impracticable in the idea. I add this note for the scientific critic, who might otherwise be disposed to carp at my imaginary, but strictly appropriate, mode of treatment.

† For simplicity's sake I omit for the present all mention of "Harmonic Upper Partials," which in practice would slightly interfere with this result, but will be explained further on.

these organs is connected with a certain number of separate nerve-fibres. When the various stimulations thus excited are communicated to the auditory centre, they are there cognized as differences in *Pitch;* the high tones being produced by undulations which recur with very great frequency, and the low ones by those which perform a smaller number of vibrations per second. In short, as a simple illustration, if we set the siren in motion, when the air first rushes through the holes with a comparatively small number of escapes per second, a very low note is recognized by the ear; as the rapidity of motion increases, and consequently the frequency of undulation becomes greater, the note is recognized as higher and higher; when the rapidity becomes immense, the note produces the effect which we call shrillness; and when the number of undulations per second exceeds some 38,000, it passes the limit of hearing altogether, probably because we have no special organ so arranged as to vibrate in sympathy with undulations of such extreme rapidity.

And now, for clearness' sake, before we pass on, let us restate from the subjective side the results at which we have arrived from the objective side. *Loudness* is independent of the organ affected: it is the result of intensity of stimulation alone; it varies with the amplitude of the air-waves, irrespective of their frequency or recurrence. All other varieties in sound depend upon the organ affected. *Noises* are the concomitants of stimulation of fibres having their terminals in the outer portion of the labyrinth; they are excited by irregular and non-periodic agitations of the air.

Musical Tones are the concomitants of stimulation of fibres having their terminals in the cochlea; they are excited by regular and periodic vibrations of certain definite frequencies. *Pitch* depends upon the particular fibre of the cochlea affected; of these, some vibrate in sympathy with undulations having slow periods, and produce low tones,—others vibrate in sympathy with undulations having rapid periods, and produce high tones. There are two other subjective phenomena of sound which have not yet been accounted for by reference to their objective counterparts in the air-waves: namely, the *Quality* or *Timbre* of different instruments; and *Note*, or the relation to one another of the different tones composing the Octave. These, however, will best be considered at a later period, when we come to investigate the subject of Musical Tones.

Though the rapid résumé I have here given of the physical nature of Hearing has demanded somewhat more space than has been accorded to the mechanism of any other sense, it must be remembered that I have only dealt with such points as are absolutely necessary for the comprehension of our present subject, the Æsthetic Feelings, and my brief summing up must not be mistaken for an attempt to set forth the true bearings of the question in its wider intellectual aspects. For fuller details the reader must be referred to the luminous and exhaustive work of Helmholtz. With this slight caution against misapprehension, we may pass on to our more proper subject.

§ 4. *General Emotional Phenomena of Hearing.*

It was noted above that the auditory nerve is only exposed to the pains of excessive action, or fatigues, and to the pleasures of gentle and normal stimulation. Let us examine a few in order.

Loudness we saw to be the subjective concomitant of excessive stimulation. Accordingly all loud and violent noises give rise to painful feelings of considerable acuteness. Thunder, the roar of a cannon, the din of steam-hammers, the whir of machinery, produce this effect. If the noise is peculiarly shrill, as in the shriek of a steam-whistle, or the screaming of parrots, the waste of tissue seems to be more intense, and the resulting feeling more unpleasant. Though these stimulations can be endured for a very few seconds, yet if long continued they so waste the tissues as to become unbearable. Certain jerky and intermittent sounds, of unpleasant intensity, such as that produced by scraping a gritty pencil over a slate, have a more special and jarring effect. This is probably due to the fact that the nerve-centres, fibres, and terminals have short intervals of repair allowed them during the intermission of the stimulant; and it is known that nerves are most sensitive to new stimulations, any continuance of excitation soon deadening their sensibility. Accordingly, in these cases, the very sensitive nerve-matter is assailed after each reparation by the violent stimulant, just at the moment when its excitability is greatest. This point will receive further illustration when we come to consider the unpleasant effects of dissonance. Even the ordinary hum of voices in a school-room, or the din of a crowded street where heavy drays rumble over rough pavements, becomes annoying when long endured, and often results in temporary deafness.

On the other hand, mere sound, when not too intense, is pleasurable as a stimulant after the oppressive silence of night or solitude. In the stillness of evening, the dipping of oars on the water, the ripple of the waves among the reeds, and the gentle hum of insects, are all agreeable reliefs. In the country, the cawing of rooks, the bleating of sheep, the lowing of cows, the murmur of the stream, are pleasant in the absence of other distracting noises. Of course, complex emotional and poetical associations come in to disturb the certainty of these instances; but it must be remembered that we lay great stress in such cases upon the *gentleness* of the sounds, as in the purling brook, the whispering zephyr, and the drowsy murmur of the humble bee:—that is to say, we recognize as important the fact that these irritants do not exceed the limits of perfectly normal stimulation. "Gentle" is the stock epithet of the poets for all these pleasant sounds of country life. Church bells, heard at a distance, are agreeable; at close quarters they become intolerable. When walking alone in the fields, we often hum or whistle, to relieve the monotony of silence; a brook by the side of our path, or the noise of ploughing, mowing, or thrashing in the neighbourhood, does away with this necessity. In almost all these cases we see that the pleasure is more or less distinctly æsthetic, and in a few of them it rises indisputably into that class.

When we progress to the human vocal organs, we notice

that those voices which are loud, shrill, and harsh, are unpleasant, while those which only stimulate our nerves of hearing within the normal limits are graceful and pretty. If they abound in musical tones, a more distinctly æsthetic element is imported, the explanation of which belongs to a later stage. Rough and jerky laughter displeases us; the "silvery" character of its opposite is a poetical commonplace. Languages which contain numerous gutturals and trilled letters make the greatest demands upon the auditory structures; aspirates and simple mutes are less objectionable; but vowels yield pure musical tones. Hence these differences are of great importance in Poetry. Highly vocalized lines are the most musical, while those containing many gutturals and treble combinations of consonants can only be admitted when intended as imitative of some rugged or harsh element in the idea expressed.

All the emotional phenomena thus grouped together show themselves to be higher in the æsthetic scale than those which we formerly examined; because they require for their perception more exercise of the intellectual faculty of attention, and are thus seen to consist of slighter and less discernible waves of pleasure and pain. Coarse and uneducated nerves cannot observe the unpleasantness of rough voices and harsh laughter; still greater discrimination is requisite for the perception of relative smoothness or ruggedness in Italian and German; while only a very attentive and highly cultivated ear can thoroughly appreciate the delicate modulation in a sentence of Burke, or the sonorous periods of Demosthenes and Cicero.

These last considerations lead us up to the first and simplest of the modes of sound which is regularly employed for a definite æsthetic purpose in works of art.

§ 5. *Rhythm.*

As we walk along the road, we sometimes amuse ourselves by touching every post, treading upon every second flag, or striking our stick against every lamp post. If for any reason we are obliged to leave out one of the series, or to desist from want of the objects in question, a slight blank is felt, which is very faintly unpleasant. The nervous system has put itself into a position of expectancy, and is ready for the appropriate discharge at the right moment. If the opportunity for the discharge is wanting, the gathered energy has to dissipate itself by other channels, which involves a certain amount of conflict and waste. In the instances cited above we should probably relieve our feelings by snapping our fingers, kicking a stone, or twirling round our stick, respectively.

The due recurrence of all such periodic actions is pleasant, because the organs then perform their functions at the exact moment of expectation. An organic rhythm is set up, and the actions correspond with it. In dances, especially such as waltzes, polkas, and galops, where the rhythm is constant, we see the simplest conscious utilization of the pleasure arising from this measured recurrence. When once we have mastered the first difficulty of learning the step, the easy mechanical nature of the periodic motion gives us abundant muscular exercise in the form most nearly approaching the æsthetic enjoyments. A false step of our partner or a mistake of our own gives us an unpleasant jar, and may entirely upset the harmonious action of the limbs for a few minutes. Of course only a small part of the pleasure derived from dancing can be set down to this cause; but that it is a real element in the enjoyment is distinctly shewn by our preference for "a good partner," merely as such.

Now, what the rhythm of the dance is to our muscular energies, the rhythm of poetry and music is to the ear. Its main constituent as a pleasure is the regularity of its recurrence, and the consequent possibility of relaxing our attention to the accentuation or the arrangement of chords. While syllables irregularly thrown together require a certain amount of jumping from point to point in the auditory perception, syllables placed in a regular order of short and long allow us to withdraw the attention from their accent, and to expect a continuance of the same harmonious and easily followed succession. Many familiar facts concur to justify this explanation. In attempting for the first time to read a perfectly new metre, it is sometimes a few minutes before we *fall into the swing of it*, as we phrase it; that is, before our auditory apparatus accommodates itself to the new mode of recurrence. Until it has done so, we derive no pleasure from the metre, which seems meanwhile the same chaos of unmeasured sequence as ordinary prose. Again, in the early stages of verse-writing, before the ear has become thoroughly trained by practice and attention, nothing is commoner than to find schoolboys send up hexameters containing seven feet, or English heroic lines with six iambi. At that point of development the ear has not become sufficiently sensitive to notice the discrepancy; to a more cultivated hearer, the effect of the sudden intrusion is abominable. Once more, a false or unmetrical line in the midst of others comparatively smooth, has a jarring effect, like that of the false step in dancing. It upsets the organic rhythm which has already established itself. On the other hand, if a few stanzas of poetry are printed as prose, we are put off our guard; we do not expect the metrical recurrence, and we may consequently read several lines before the ear begins to detect the regularity of the accent or quantity. We may therefore conclude that the æsthetic pleasure of metre depends upon the existence of an expectant state, realized in the auditory apparatus as a recurrent organic rhythm of nascent stimulation: while the æsthetic discomfort of bad versification depends upon the breach of this expectation, and consequent upsetting of the organic rhythm. In this connexion it is perhaps worth notice that almost all the greatest masters of musical expression amongst English poets have been educated in the practice of verse-composition in the dead languages, which (useless though it is as a means of general culture) possesses the solitary advantage of giving to the ear a sensitiveness to metrical accuracy hardly obtainable in any other way. This is especially noticeable in Milton, and in our great living poets, whose achievements in metrical technique far surpass anything that can be found in our earlier literature.

Of course many other sensuous and emotional factors enter into the composition of metrical pleasure, especially in those higher flights to which allusion has just been made. In the first place, lines may be highly vocalized and all disagreeable consonantal combinations rejected. This is especially desirable in anapæstic and dactylic verse, where rapidity and ease of touch are the points chiefly aimed at. Mr. Swinburne's *Dolores* is a perfect marvel of execution in this respect. Again, a great deal of intellectual pleasure may be given by an apt adaptation of metre to sense. Iambics (in English) are slow and solemn; spondees, heavy; dactyls, graceful and rapid; trochees, stirring and suitable for martial pieces. Besides the skill which may thus be shown in the choice of metre for a whole composition in accordance with its subject, great power of imitation may be exhibited in adapting even a comparatively fixed metre to a momentary emotion by slight changes in the constituent feet. Take the following two lines of the *Atys* as examples, which I have pointed for those readers who may not be already acquainted with the metre;

> "Tibi″cen ubi′ cani″t Phry″x curvo″ grave ca′lamo″;
> Ubi ca′pita Mœ″nade″s vi″ jaciu″nt hederi′geræ″."

Or these from Tennyson;

> "The long brook falling through the cloven ravine
> In *cataract after cataract* to the sea."

Or once more from the same delicate artist;

> "The great brand
> Made lightnings in the splendour of the moon,
> And flashing round and round, and *whirled in an arch*,
> Shot like a streamer of the northern morn,
> Seen where the moving isles of winter shock
> By night, with noises of the northern sea."

In all these the pleasure is partly owing to the fact that, while the balance of expectation is preserved by keeping the same number of accented syllables throughout, a very small variation is introduced with an obviously imitative purpose which at once forces itself upon the notice of the intellect. Even for mere variety's sake, without any imitative intention, some such ringing the changes is often employed with artistic effect; as in the weak cæsura of Latin hexameters, the frequent tribrachs and less common dactyls or anapæsts of Greek senarii,* and the occasional trisyllables which Shelley showed how to incorporate amongst the iambi of English blank verse. In all these cases, besides the pure rhythmical pleasure, intellectual elements are involved, which will have to be considered in a later chapter.

Under the present heading we may briefly mention the other poetical devices of rhyme and (in some classes of poetry, such as the Early English) alliteration. These likewise obviously depend for their effect upon the principle of recurrence and expectation.

* I do not include the spondees, and for a definite reason. They form really a component part of the metre. Pure iambic trimeters make a distinct species, differing materially from the ordinary senarius. The figment of grammarians, that metres begin with a pure form, and that impure feet are afterwards admitted, is the exact opposite of historical truth. Metre, being originally written by ear (and very imperfect ears, too,) is at first extremely rough and irregular. It is only by gradual refinements and tentative efforts that it becomes accommodated to the absolute requirements of the trained poet. The Latin hexameter had to pass through the various stages of Livius, Ennius, Lucretius, and Catullus, before it attained the perfect modulation of the Second Georgic. The iambics of the *Phaselus* would have proved far too troublesome for a less cultivated versifier than their author. In the present generation Mr. Swinburne has shown Englishmen for the first time that metres composed purely of trisyllabic feet are possible in their language.

After what has been said before it will hardly be necessary to point out that the various pleasures and disappointments enumerated in this section are composed of very slight emotional elements, require for their perception much trained attention and delicacy of nervous constitution, and belong consequently to the most distinctively æsthetic class. It is also clear that the pleasures arise from the maximum of stimulation with the minimum of fatigue; and that the disappointments, being due to breach of expectation and consequent upsetting of an organic rhythm, are traceable to the felt want of this harmonious species of stimulation.

§ 6. *Musical Tone.*

Several times in the course of the preceding sections allusion has been made to the pleasurableness of Musical Tones, coupled with a promise of its future explanation. At this point we now arrive. We have seen wherein these tones differ in intellectual discriminability from other sounds; we have now to explain their emotional superiority.

It was mentioned above that Musical Tones result from the periodic vibrations of an elastic or oscillatory body, and that their pitch depends upon the frequency per second of the aërial undulations so produced. It was also noticed that the mode of their perception is probably by sympathetic vibrations aroused in Corti's organs, the elastic appendages to the nerve-terminations in the cochlea. As any single pure tone can only excite such sympathetic vibrations in a single one of Corti's organs,* we not only see the reason why so large

* This, which is doubtless strictly true of absolutely simple tones, like

a number of tones are intellectually discriminable, but also why Musical Tones are in themselves, and apart from combinational effects, more pleasant to us than mere Noises. While the outer portion of the ear, which probably responds to the wide range of undulations giving rise to Noises, is constantly undergoing stimulation; each one of Corti's organs, being limited in its sympathy to a very small range of vibrations, is comparatively seldom excited by its proper irritant. Hence we may conclude that the corresponding fibre and the connected portions of the auditory centre are usually in that high state of nutrition which is the condition-precedent of pleasurable stimulation. Accordingly we find that almost all the more distinctly pleasurable sounds, such as the song of birds, the human voice, and the tones of various musical instruments, are made up of vibrations of the periodic sort.

But between the various tones so produced there exist considerable differences in emotional effect. Some are said to be rich and mellow; others, harsh and poor. Some, when sounded together, produce a consonance; others, a dissonance. In order to comprehend these differences, we must go a little deeper than we have hitherto done into the physical composition of air-waves, as well as their physiological and psychical counterparts.

If we produce upon the siren air-waves of any given frequency per second, we hear a tone subjectively recognized as

those of a siren or a tuning-fork, is interfered with in most cases by those other undulations which produce "Harmonic Upper Partials." That phenomenon, however, I persistently disregard for the present, as it merely complicates the question in hand.

being of a certain definite pitch. If we then double the frequency per second, by making the siren perform twice as many revolutions in the same time, we obtain a different tone, recognized subjectively as such, and yet standing in a certain definite relation in consciousness to the previous tone, which is expressed by saying that the second is the *Octave* of the first. If we again double the frequency of undulation, we obtain a third tone similarly recognized as the Octave of the second. And so on till the limit of audibility is reached.

If, once more, instead of doubling the number of revolutions (and consequently of vibrations) we make the siren perform three revolutions in the time in which it formerly performed two, the note will be higher in Pitch than it previously was, in a certain analogous recognisable ratio, which is known as a *Fifth.*

Similarly, we find that if the siren produces first three revolutions per second, and then four, the resulting relation of tones is known as a *Fourth.* If it first performs four revolutions per second, and then five, the relation is known as a *Major Third.* If it first performs five per second, and then six, the interval is called a *Minor Third.* Two other rather more complicated intervals (immaterial numerically to our purpose) are known as *Major* and *Minor Sixths.*

All tones which stand in these numerical relations to one another are said to have *consonant intervals.* The meaning of this term will be explained hereafter: for the present we shall adopt it as a convenient name. The eight tones which bear such relations to one another are said to form an

Octave. This, then, is the physical difference which gives rise in consciousness to the distinction between the *Notes* of the Octave.

So far we have treated both the air-waves and the tones to which they give rise as though they were perfectly simple and uncompounded. This is actually the case with a small number of air-waves which originate musical sounds, such as those of the siren or the tuning-fork. But the vast majority of vibrating bodies, like violin-strings or the human vocal organs, have been proved to produce air-waves compounded of many undulations having different frequencies; because, while the whole vibrates as a whole, various fractional parts also vibrate independently as parts. The first class may be described as *simple*, the second as *compound* wave-systems. Again, it has been shown that a compound wave-system may be analysed into its component factors by a series of resonators, each of which has been so regulated as to vibrate sympathetically with one set of undulations only, of a given frequency, amongst those which form the compound system. And, in the human ear, Corti's organs, being practically just such a series of resonators, probably analyse the whole wave-system into its various factors, so that each of them is heard as a separate and very slight tone of a recognisable pitch. Accordingly, the whole tone heard when a violin-string is set in motion is not simple and undecomposable, but is a compound of many simple tones, all of different pitch, each of which is called a *partial tone*, in contra-distinction to the *compound tone* which results from their combination. A good musical ear can easily recognise these partial tones, and discriminate between one loudest and lowest note (produced by the vibration of the whole, and known as the *prime tone*) and other less loud and higher ones, called the *upper partials*. Lastly, these various sets of waves with different periods which compose the compound wave-system may or may not stand towards that largest class of undulations which give rise to the prime-tone in the numerical relations given above as constituting the consonant intervals: and, accordingly, may or may not produce tones standing in the relation of musical intervals to the prime-tone. In the former case they are said to be *harmonic*, in the latter case, *inharmonic*, upper partials.

Before we proceed to examine the reasons for the pleasure derived from consonance of tones and the objectionable nature of dissonance, we may notice one æsthetic application of the above principles which can conveniently be made at the present stage. We have already seen that musical tones are more agreeable than mere noises, because, while the nervous apparatus for the perception of the latter receives frequent stimulation, each portion of the nervous apparatus for the perception of the former is comparatively seldom stimulated, and is therefore usually in that high state of nutrition which is the necessary condition for pleasurable excitement. Accordingly, to carry the same argument a step further, a stimulant which would affect a large number of these special organs would afford greater pleasure than one which affected a single organ and its connected fibres alone. Now the tones produced by simple uncompounded undulations, having a single pitch—like those of tuning-forks—can only arouse a sympathetic vibration in a single one of Corti's organs: and we find, as might be expected, that such undulations produce a tone not used in Music, and characterised by its *poverty* and *dullness*. On the other hand, the tones produced by wave-systems compounded of many individual sets of undulations, each having its own frequency—like those of violin-strings—ought naturally to excite sympathetically many of Corti's organs, with their connected fibres, and to be cognised as a mass of sounds, differing in pitch: and we find that these are the wave-systems most employed in Music, as yielding tones noted for their *richness* and *fullness*—expressions which well describe the actual physiological effect. This result is only interfered with by the singular phenomenon of dissonance, to which we must next proceed.

Up to this point we have treated of air-waves as though a number of systems could be propagated side by side with each other through the atmosphere without mutual interference. But this is not really the case. If two series of simple undulations are produced upon the siren, it is found that in certain cases the waves mutually interfere in such a manner that they at one time reinforce and at another cancel one another. The reason of this is that the crests and troughs of the waves are alternated in such an order that occasionally (at fixed intervals) two crests or two troughs coincide, when of course the resulting undulation is of greater amplitude, and at others a crest and a trough coincide, in which case they neutralise one another. Now whenever this phenomenon of interference in the waves occurs with moderately long intervals, the ear is conscious of each separate interruption of the tone, and each subsequent reinforcement. Such alternations of sound are called *Beats*. But if the intervals between the interferences are very slight, then the ear at last fails to recognise the separate beats as such, and is merely conscious of that rough and discordant sound which we call a *dissonance*. As a matter of physics, it has been shown that all orders of undulations produce with one another interferences (and consequently dissonances due to these minute beats) unless they stand to one another in the numerical relations of frequency which correspond to the consonant intervals of Music.

But why should these interferences produce unpleasant sensations? The solution of this question is the key to the whole difficulty of harmony and discord: and that solution we owe to Helmholtz. It was stated above that the ear is one of the organs whose repair is carried on at the most rapid rate. After every stimulation the fibres and nerve-centres are quickly put back into the proper state of nutrition for performing their ordinary functions. But the intermittent character of the stimulation in air-waves subject to interferences taxes the structures to the uttermost. For it is a common experience that continued stimulation of a nerve deadens it after a short time to the action of the stimulus; while intermission of the stimulation gives time for a renewal of the nervous excitability, and a consequent liability to fresh stimulation. Accordingly, the rapid alternation of irritation and repair set up by air-waves whose mutual interference produces rapidly-recurring beats, is highly destructive of nervous tissue. At the very moment when the sensibility of the nerve is renewed after the last preceding shock, a second and a third shock come to waste its newly-recovered strength. We have already seen that rapid alternation of stimulation in the tactile corpuscles produced the jarring sensation of gritty touch; that a similar rapid alternation in the case of the auditory nerves in the vestibule produced the unpleasant thrill of a pencil scratched over a slate; and we shall see hereafter in examining the sense of sight that the rapid alternation of light and shadow in a flickering candle or an intermittent series of electric sparks affects in like manner the optic apparatus. In passing beside a fence through which the sunlight flickers alternately between the palings, we have all experienced the unpleasant effect of such intermission. So, whenever two series of aerial undulations interfere with one another in such a manner as to produce alternate reinforcement and cancelling, with rapid rates of recurrence, the effect upon the auditory nervous system is that of severe and intermittent stimulation, wastefully attacking the fibres and end-organs concerned, and cognized in consciousness as a special form of discomfort called a dissonance.

Not only can simple series of air-waves thus interfere with one another, but so also can the several members of those compound wave-systems which we saw to be the objective counterparts of musical tones possessing harmonic upper partials. Indeed, as a rule, dissonances are more often produced by interferences between the lesser members of each series than between the main undulations which correspond to their prime tones. And as all orders of undulations, except those which stand to one another in the numerical relations which underlie the consonant intervals, have been shown both by mathematical calculation and physical experiment to produce such interferences, it results that only those ratios which yield the consonant tones can be employed together for æsthetic effect. They, alone, when conjoined, continuously and harmoniously stimulate the auditory fibres; all other combinations yield that intermittent stimulation which is cognised in consciousness as discord.

Finally, the component members of a single compound wave system, yielding a tone with upper partials, may produce such interferences with one another; in which case the tone itself is cognised as unmusical, rough, or braying.

We left open for awhile, above, the question as to what was the objective fact which underlay the distinction of *timbre* or *quality* between tones of the same apparent pitch, sounded upon different instruments or different human voices. It will be seen from what has been said hitherto that this distinction really depends upon the number and character of the harmonic (or inharmonic) upper partials which each possesses; or, to put the same fact objectively, upon the various periodic frequencies of the various members composing the compound wave-system. While in any two such cases the periodic frequency of that dominant member of the system which yields the prime tone is the same, and affects sympathetically the same one of Corti's organs, (or else we would not regard the two as possessing the same pitch) the number and frequency of the various minor component members which yield the harmonic (or inharmonic) upper partials may be very different, and so give rise to sympathetic vibrations in different units of Corti's organs, and be consequently differentially cognised in consciousness. The distinction thus originated is called *quality* or *timbre.* I need hardly add that those qualities are agreeable which stimulate the largest number of fibres with the greatest freedom from mutually-produced interferences; and those qualities objectionable which stimulate fewest fibres or produce mutual interferences. The former class are said to be *rich,* the latter *poor* and *harsh* respectively.

Lastly, we see that these emotional effects are still more minute in character and still more difficult of discrimination than those that we have hitherto examined; and we consequently decide that they stand highest of all the auditory class in the æsthetic scale.

§ 7. *Music.*

It is not my intention to enter into the deeper questions of musical composition, partly because I am not qualified by musical tastes to do so, and partly because Music, except in those elementary phases which have been hitherto treated, does not largely enter in the ideal form into the composition of Poetry, which is the ultimate end of our present inquiry. It may be well, however, to glance briefly at some few points which especially demand our attention.

In the first place, just as the principle by which (though

unconsciously) we are guided in the choice of certain modifications of the human voice, and certain reeds or strings, for musical purposes, is that they produce the maximum of stimulation with the minimum of fatigue or waste; so, too, in the combination of these elements, the same end is held steadily in view. A chord consists of a combination of tones, none of which produces a dissonance with another, either in primes or partials. Such chords are then placed together in that systematic order which yields a musical phrase, that is, a consciously-felt harmonious pleasurable stimulation, in the complex total as well as the several elements. And, in a complete composition, such a rational and intelligible sequence of phrases is sought after as will give the whole a definite completeness as a single work, not a mere collection of chords. This can only be done by combining the various parts upon a regular plan, which involves an immense deal of previous association, and, probably, a certain amount of conventional arrangement.

As an assistance in attaining such an intelligible order, musical tones are not permitted to vary indefinitely in duration, but are arranged in a definite scale of length, each note lasting double the time of the next below, and half the time of the next above. Hence we are enabled to arrange them in various combinations, which give varying degrees of prominence to one tone or another. We can employ chiefly semibreves, minims, and crotchets, to produce slow and solemn music; or we can use mainly the shorter notes, and produce rapid and easy tunes. Moreover, these differences in duration and their ratios to one another are readily recognised by the ear, so that we can perceive a certain orderly arrangement in the time as well as the tune, and an adaptation of the one to the other, which appeals to our intellectual faculties and our love of symmetry.

But the great mass of pleasurable feeling aroused by Music is undoubtedly due to its power of suggesting and stimulating the various complex emotions. *Why* these emotions yield us pleasure is a question that must be left for a later chapter; but we may well enquire here how Music has acquired this power of arousing them. It is a well-known fact that mere collocations of sound, without words or other interpretation, will rouse martial enthusiasm, quicken religious feeling, or bring tears into the eyes of thousands. To account for these effects is difficult, but we may perhaps see how they are brought about if we follow up the growth of such emotional associations from their simplest germs.

The high and low tones respectively are the natural expressions of different passing emotions both in man and other animals. We get the earliest case in mere shouts and cries which express joy, surprise, anger, or surliness, without forethought or concert. A step above these are the dance of victory with its accompanying song of triumph; or the wailing and funereal cries, which are regularly planned and consciously carried out. Such performances may be accompanied by chanted words, in which case the varying ideas implied by them will have their varying but natural emotional expression, changing with every change of thought. In this way a first beginning will be made, by which certain modes of sound become associated with certain phases of emotion. As music becomes more conscious and more differentiated, attempts will spontaneously be made to suit the time and tune more definitely to the idea expressed. Instrumental aid will also be called in. The hollow timbrel is fitted for slow funereal marches; the tinkling cymbals express the joy of victory and welcome the conquerors home. More extensive imitations of emotional expression next arise. The more delicate affections, grief, tenderness, rapture, have appropriate tones, which can be combined with words that eke out the half-expressed idea. Rapid transitions produce one distinct effect; slow rhythm another. Songs of purely musical character thus grow up slowly out of the monotonous chants and spontaneous recitatives of savages. Instrumental music is similarly developed from the rude clamour of the tom-tom, the rattle, and the gong. Artificial association does the rest. Certain combinations have always been employed in connexion with particular phases of thought, and recall them at once. Gregorian music has always been heard in dim cathedrals or on Sabbath evenings, and so, besides its natural solemnity, revives the memories of those sacred scenes. The tripping measure of dance-music suggests the gay throngs with which it is most closely connected in thought. Thus we have gradually come to recognise certain combinations of time and tune as specially adapted to sacred, processional, martial, tender, or gay subjects. These, again, subdivide into more special classes, recalling more special emotions. In the oratorio, the subject alone suggests the extraneous association. In the opera, dress, gesture, language, and action, all aid the realization of the musical import. Here then we are able to form numerous other emotional and classical associations, all partly natural in their ground-work, but all owing something to the conventional interpretation that we learn to put upon them. At last, by all these various steps, we reach that final power of receiving special emotional stimulation from sounds alone which is illustrated in such compositions as the Lieder ohne Wörte.*

Expression in composition depends upon an intimate knowledge of these various effects and a vast repertory of combinations suitable for their production. Expression in execution depends upon realization of the composer's meaning. The performer must intellectually grasp the idea that was in the mind of his composer, and must aid its development by exerting all his technical skill in rendering. This can only adequately be done by minute discrimination of the faintest emotional shades in touch, cadence, and timbre, combined with perfect delicacy of fingering, or thorough command over the muscles of song. It is just this power of putting himself in harmony with the spirit of a great master, and reproducing in faithful representation his innermost conception, that above all other points distinguishes the true artiste from the mere brilliant executionist. The one plays and sings the notes, the other plays and sings the idea.

And if the perception of harmony and discord in simple

* For the relation of Music to natural expression see Mr. Herbert Spencer's Essay on the "Origin and Function of Music."

combinations of two tones demands a comparatively high order of emotional discriminativeness, it is immediately obvious that these higher and successively higher combinations of re-representative elements require for their appreciation a successively minuter and more delicate discriminativeness, besides a deeper emotional and intellectual nature. Hence they are amply entitled to the first place in the æsthetic scale of Hearing, if not, indeed, in the whole hierarchy of the senses. Music is claimed by its admirers as the highest of the directly presentative arts, and surpassed by Poetry alone, the absolutely ideal and representative form of æsthetic gratification.

CHAPTER VII.

SIGHT.

§ 1. *Æsthetic Importance of Sight.*

THE enormous majority of æsthetic objects appeal to the sense of Sight, and it must accordingly be placed first of the senses in the æsthetic hierarchy. This will seem a hard saying to the musically-minded, but a little consideration will justify it to any unprejudiced thinker. It must be remembered that only a few natural sounds, such as the song of birds, the hum of insects, and the murmur of water, are æsthetically beautiful; while, besides the artistic device of rhythm, only a single art—that of Music—is based upon the sense of Hearing; and it adds comparatively few ideal elements to Poetry. But Sight yields us numerous gratifications from natural objects of all sorts, as well as endless pleasures of æsthetic effect in manufactured articles, keramic, textile, and general; while, amongst the higher arts, three principal ones, Painting, Sculpture, and Architecture, are founded upon it alone; and immensely the larger part of the ideal sensuous elements in Poetry are of visual origin, in one of the modes, as form or colour.

A brief enumeration of some among these various objects

will perhaps aid us in estimating the importance for our present subject of the sense which we have now to attack. Amongst natural æsthetic products owing their beauty to visual qualities we may mention, in the organic world, bright-hued flowers, green leaves, plants or trees, and coloured foliage; sea anemones and other brilliant radiata; shells of mollusca or articulata; butterflies, beetles, and moths; birds of bright or delicate plumage; and many graceful or beautiful mammals, such as the antelope, the zebra, the tiger, and the hare. Here, too, we must place the beauty of human beings, man or woman, adult or child. In the inorganic world, we have gems and precious stones: marble, amber, jet, and porphyry; the various metals, especially gold and silver; with all the coloured woods, stones, sands, and clays. Amongst effects of light in a more transitory form may be reckoned the rainbow and the hues of sunset, the solar spectrum, the dew-drop, and iridescence generally on water, ice, crystals, or thin plates of any transparent substance. We have direct light in the sun, fixed stars, fire-flies, glow-worms, and the phosphorescence of the sea. Amongst larger collections of natural objects we may notice woods, valleys, mountains, rivers, lakes, glaciers, rocks, waterfalls, the stormy ocean, the blue expanse of heaven, and the autumn tints upon the forest. All these, combined, go to make up what we call scenery. To this list we must add the artificial products which man has wrought out of these natural objects or agencies. Beginning with the feathers, shells, and pebbles of the savage, we go up through all the grades of dress, dyed cloths, purple and fine linen, silk, lace, furs, jewellery, and embroidery. Similarly with upholstery, from the simple rushes and wooden bench of primitive royalty to the Turkey carpets, pomegranate wall papers, mahogany tables, marble mantelpieces, lace curtains, and satin coverings of modern civilized life. Pottery and domestic utensils, too, have passed from the rough clay pipkin and the rudely-carved calabash, to Greek and Etruscan vases, Palissy and Wedgwood ware, the goblets of Cellini and the many-hued Venetian glass. Architecture has grown from the wattled hut and the wooden Ionian cottage to Corinthian columns, Roman domes, Gothic cathedrals, and Indian temples. It has superadded to natural scenery the further charms of the towering fortress, the ruined castle, the venerable abbey, the village spire, the bridge spanning the cataract, and the cottage perched upon the crags ; all of which give the sense of human occupation, past or present, and relieve the solitude of unpeopled nature. Side by side with these, cultivation has introduced the close-shaven lawn, the trim croft, the hedges and walls which impart individuality to each element of the scene; the hay-ricks, the apple-orchards, the vineyard, and the waving corn-fields. Finally, we have the more distinctly æsthetic arts of Painting and Sculpture, which imitate and emulate all these, besides appealing indirectly to the various complex emotions, and so inducing to the fullest extent that compound sensuous and emotional thrill which we know in its synthetic totality as artistic pleasure.

With such a vast repertory as this, Sight may well claim to take first rank in the æsthetic order of the senses.

§ 2. *Æther-waves and the Organ for their Perception.*

Besides the atmospheric air which continually surrounds us, modern science teaches us to assume that there exists everywhere a much subtler and apparently imponderable fluid, known as the Æther, which we figure to ourselves as filling not only the vast interstellar spaces, but also the minute interstices between the molecules and atoms of all ponderable bodies, the gases of the atmosphere itself included. Of the true nature of this Æther we know nothing with certainty: indeed, we may regard it rather as a hypothetical expression which enables us to comprehend certain orders of facts than as a real and indubitable existence. But whatever may be the doubts which rest over the nature of the Æther, we can feel quite sure of the reality of many manifestations which we can only formulate to ourselves as modes of motion in this imponderable and all-pervading fluid. As such, then, we shall unhesitatingly regard them, remembering that the truth of our explanations is in no way bound up with that of the theory in terms of which they are at present necessarily expressed: for the proved and measureable energies which we thus figure to our minds will remain equally real, and every mathematical formula with reference to them will be equally correct, whatever may be the ultimate fate of our present mode of representation.*

* I use this doubtful language for fear of those strainers at gnats, who can swallow the whole material universe, but refuse the one item of Æther. It is amusing to see the naïveté with which most scientific men (who are not metaphysicians) accept unhesitatingly the existence of air, while they plume themselves upon their caution in using hypothetical terms with refer-

The Æther, like all other fluids, is capable of being set in rhythmical or oscillatory motion, so as to produce recurrent undulations. It is not largely affected, however, by those greater oscillations which produce the air-waves, cognized in consciousness as sound. It is true that air-waves as they die away give up their energy at last to the Æther; but the ordinary and best-known undulations of the latter have a different origin. The motion which usually produces this effect upon the imponderable fluid is that rapid and minute vibration of material particles which takes place when their temperature is considerably raised, and the Æther-waves thus generated are infinitely smaller and quicker than those of the air. Any body whose particles are in this state of rapid vibration (commonly induced by chemical combination with other substances) impinges upon the surrounding Æther and sets up in it a series of undulations which spread in every direction in straight lines. The particular nature of these undulations and their differences from those air-waves which constitute the objective basis of sound, need not here be entered into. They do not concern our immediate subject, and they can be found in any treatise on Physical Optics. All that we need at present notice is their physiological effect, and the mode of their final psychical perception.

If we warm a piece of iron, short of red-heat, in a darkened room, and then hold it a few inches from the face, we are

ence to Æther. As though all forms of matter, ponderable or imponderable, were not equally mere symbols of unknown realities or possibilities, all alike revealed to us simply through their effects upon the human senses. We know just as much about air as we do about Æther, and no more: that is to ay, exactly nothing.

conscious of a peculiar sensation in our cheeks, which we name heat. This sensation is produced by waves of Æther, which attack the nerve-terminations of those fibres, distributed over the whole body, whose office is to inform us of changes in the temperature of our skin.* The undulations of the Æther may be supposed to set up corresponding undulations in the terminals or adjacent tissues, and the stimulus thus received is transmitted by the fibres to the brain. The Æther-waves so cognized are comparatively slow in their rates of oscillation, though many times more rapid than those of the atmosphere which give rise to sound. But there are other Æther-waves far quicker than these. If we replace the iron in the fire, its rate of vibration becomes much more rapid, and when we again withdraw it, we find not only that the sensation of heat is intensified, but also that a new sensation arises, localized in our eyes. The iron has become red-hot, and now yields, besides the first and slower class of undulations which we knew as heat, another and more rapid class of undulations which we know as light. The mode of action in the first case is a very familiar one. We know that whenever the slower Æther-waves, which we distinguish by the name of Radiant Heat, fall upon any object, they set up in it sympathetic vibrations; which we call Absorbed Heat. It is quite intelligible that these vibrations should affect the terminations of the thermal nerves, and so give rise to the sensation of Heat. But the mode of action in the second

* We assume the existence of special thermal fibres, because it is difficult otherwise to bring the case of heat and cold under the general principle of specific energies. Another explanation may, however, be discovered hereafter.

case is more special, and it resides in a more specialized organ,—the eye. This, indeed, is quite what we might expect. The varying degrees of temperature are of the utmost importance to animal life, which they affect directly; and even very low animal organisms are accordingly provided with nervous structures sensitive to heat and cold. But the more rapid Æther-waves which we cognize as Light, though all-important to vegetables, do not produce so immediate results upon animal life; and the various indications which they yield are only valuable with the help of a comparatively complex system of organic co-ordination—known subjectively as *intellect*—in the development of which system they bear the chief part. Accordingly, we find the organ of Sight wanting in the lowest animals, only slightly developed in the intermediate classes, and attaining an advanced state of perfection in the higher articulata and the vertebrates alone. And side by side with this advance in visual adaptation we find a general advance in intelligence. We need only concern ourselves here with that particular form of the organ of Sight which is found in man.

The essential portions of the human eye are two in number: first, an outer or conducting portion, by which the Æther-waves are received and converged upon the nervous structure; and, second, an inner sensitive portion, where the waves impinge upon the nerve-terminations and set up action in the fibres. The most important part of the external eye is the crystalline lens, a viscid body capable of converging Æther-waves upon the sensitive background, in the same manner as the ordinary glass lenses used by opticians. But, owing to its semi-liquid consistency, it is possible to alter its shape and focus by a muscular contraction so as to converge at will Æther-waves from different sources at varying distances upon a given point behind it, and thus to save the necessity for many separate lenses, which would have to be used if the material employed were solid.* The inner or sensitive portion consists of the retina, a net-work of nerve-terminations, whose principal organs, known as the *rods* and *cones*, are spread like a piece of tessellated pavement in close ranks over the back of the eye. Their exact nature or functions are not perfectly understood: we may regard it as probable, however, that the Æther-waves set up in them some kind of sympathetic vibration which communicates its disturbance to the fibres of the optic nerve. At any rate, we know that these terminations are the most delicate and the most minutely discriminative in the whole body; and there are many reasons for supposing that they consist of specially unstable nerve-substance, so arranged as to be easily affected by almost infinitesimal incident energies, like those of the quicker ætherial undulations. Each point upon the retina corresponds to a particular spot in the visual field; and when nervous action is set up in any such point, the resulting sensation is regarded as having its objective origin in the corresponding external spot. The nature and cause of this connexion is a question belonging to the analysis of our intellectual faculties: it must merely be accepted as a datum in the science of Æsthetics.

* All questions as to the mode of convergence belong simply to Physical Optics, that is, the objective science of Æther-waves and their transforma-

§ 3. *Varieties of Æther-waves and their Equivalents in Consciousness.*

So far we have only recognized that broadest distinction between Æther-waves upon which are based the widely-different sensations of Light and Heat. We have next to enquire what are the minor varieties of undulation, and how they are separately cognized by the organ of vision. Here again we must necessarily speak with great brevity, referring the reader for details to special works upon the subject.

If we pass a pencil of Æther-waves, proceeding from any incandescent body, through a prism in a darkened room, we split up the pencil into a number of separate series of undulations, varying in their rapidity of oscillation, just as we saw that the air-waves which produce sound, varied according to the rate of vibration in the generating body. We find, too, that the waves arrange themselves in a regular order, beginning with those slowest ones which produce heat, and ending with the most rapid of all. If we project the divided pencil upon a screen, we can measure the number of varieties; and when we do so, we are conscious, visually, of a belt of coloured bands, beginning with red and ending with violet. If, beyond the red band, we insert a thermo-electric pile, we find that the slowest waves which produce heat are mostly concentrated upon a region outside the coloured bands on that side; and if we test the other end, beyond the violet, with certain chemically-prepared surfaces,

tions : it would be impossible to treat that subject even cursorily in a work like the present.

we find that the opposite class of very rapid waves, possessing great chemical activity, are mostly concentrated upon a corresponding region outside the bands on the contrary side. Between these two points we find the various colours arranged in visible order. Hence we conclude that the slowest and the most rapid undulations alike fail to affect the nerves of the eye; but that the intermediate classes of waves fall upon the retina and there excite differential sensations. By what mechanism they do so is our next question. This we are enabled to answer with great probability by Young's theory of the perception of colour, which may now be regarded almost in the light of a proved law.

We may suppose that all over the surface of the retina nervous terminations are closely packed, belonging to three orders which correspond to three classes of fibres and their connected central organs. Each order of terminations vibrates in sympathy with a system of Æther-waves possessing a limited though widely varying rate of oscillation only. From the stimulation of those in sympathy with the slowest (visible) waves arises the sensation of red. From the stimulation of those in sympathy with waves having a medium rate of oscillation arises the sensation of green. From the stimulation of those in sympathy with the quickest (visible) waves arises the sensation of violet. All other sensations of colour are due to combinations of these in different degrees of intensity. Stimulation of all three simultaneously produces the feeling of whiteness. Stimulation of the red and green produces the sensation called yellow: of the green and violet, that called blue: of the violet and red, that called purple. Hence the visible shape of any object depends upon the number and position of the points in the retina affected by it: its colour depends upon the class of nervous terminations stimulated; and this last point, again, depends upon the rapidity of the Æther-waves which impinge upon the particular portion. So that, in the eye as in the ear, differences of sensation are ultimately explicable as due to differences in the several structures involved.*

It is obvious from what has been said above that an ordinary pencil of Æther-waves consists of many systems possessing all the various rates of oscillation, from the slowest to the most rapid. In the method of sifting by means of a prism, adopted in our illustration, all these various systems are separated from one another, so that in one place we get the slowest or heat-rays; in another the somewhat quicker or red rays; next to them again, with increasing rapidity, the orange, yellow, green, blue, and violet rays; and last of all, the quickest or ultra-violet rays. But there is another and commoner mode of sifting the component wave-systems of compound ætherial undulations, by what is called interference. In order to understand this method, which gives their distinctive proper colours to all material objects, we must first examine very briefly the simpler case of reflexion.

When a pencil of compound ætherial undulations falls upon a perfectly smooth and polished opaque surface, it is

* The number of separate kinds of terminations must be accepted as purely conjectural. The ordinary explanation is that given in the text, but the real numbers may be much greater.

not analyzed into its component factors, but is turned back again in its totality (at least so far as concerns its visible constituents) at an angle equal to that of its original incidence. Such a pencil is said to be reflected. If, into our darkened room, we admit a single pencil of Æther-waves, and then project it upon a mirror so as to return the reflected ray upon our eyes, we obtain an image as strong as we should get by placing our eyes in the direct path of the pencil. The rays may be all returned, if the reflecting surface is an (ideally) perfect one; or they may be partly returned and partly transmitted; or they may be returned in portion only, and the remainder absorbed by the body.

This, then, is what happens when the opaque surface upon which the pencil falls is perfectly smooth and polished. But most ordinary objects are not so uniform as the mirror. They consist of innumerable minor surfaces, each of which receives and reflects the Æther-waves at a different angle. Nor do they all reflect the total beam in all its constituents alike. Some orders of undulations are occasionally absorbed by an interference similar to that which we noticed in the case of air-waves. If, instead of the mirror, we place in the path of the pencil a particular piece of prepared silk, (I purposely avoid misleading terms which already involve the fact of colour-perception) we shall find that the pencil is no longer reflected in its totality; only the rays of a particular rapidity—say in this case those which produce the sensation of redness—are cast off by the silk; and even these are not directly reflected in a single pencil, but scattered in every direction through the room. Now all opaque surfaces thus scatter the Æther-waves that fall upon them, sometimes returning them all, in which case the surface is said to be white; sometimes absorbing many and returning a few, but all in equal proportions, in which case it is called grey; sometimes returning those of one or two orders only, the remainder being neutralized by interference, in which case the object is said to be red, green, blue, or yellow, according to the kind of waves which it reflects; and sometimes absorbing all the rays, in which case the surface is said to be black.

The principal object subserved by our eyes is the recognition of such dispersed and reflected light. It is the Æther-waves thus cast off in every direction from the surfaces of material bodies which have had the main share in the development of the visual organs. Before the introduction of fires, candles, lucifer matches, and gas-lamps, the sun and the fixed stars were almost the only objects which could affect the nascent or developed vision with direct light. To become cognizant of these distant bodies could not be of any practical importance to the differentiating organisms. But all the various terrestrial objects around us are perpetually casting off waves from their surfaces in every direction, which fall upon the nerve-terminations of the eye, and yield special indications of form and colour, immediately translated by the intellect into their corresponding tactual terms. And this probably explains the reason why the eye is only sensible to the middle or visible rays of the spectrum, and not to the two extreme bands. The slowest or heat rays, besides the fact that they do not pass readily through the crystalline lens, are mostly absorbed by the surfaces upon which they fall, instead of being reflected like the light-rays: and the quickest or ultrà-violet rays, besides being absorbed by the crystalline lens in the production of fluorescence, are probably present in very small numbers in dispersed light. At any rate, confining ourselves to the visible portion of the spectrum, we may conclude with great probability that the existence of special nerve-terminations for the perception of the various colours is due to the sifting of total solar Æther-waves by most terrestrial surfaces, and the consequent dispersed reflexion of different systems of undulations from different bodies in the environment. As any tendency which might arise towards the establishment of such differentially-affected structures would be obviously for the advantage of the organism, by giving it more specialized information with regard to food, enemies, or other relatively-important facts in its surroundings, it would of course be perpetuated and increased through the joint action of heredity and selection, so as to produce at last that minutely-constructed and highly-discriminative organ, the mammalian and human eye.

With this brief and somewhat diagrammatic *résumé* of the mode of action in vision we pass on to our more proper subject, the pleasures and pains derived from the eye.

§ 4. *General Emotional Phenomena of Sight.*

The eye, like the ear, is not ordinarily exposed to any destructive disintegrative action, nor to violent and long-intermitted stimulation. Hence its pains are chiefly those of exhaustion and fatigue, in the whole or a part of the nervous structures; while its pleasures are chiefly those of normal and harmonious stimulation, occurring after comparatively short periods of sufficient repair and nutrition. We will briefly examine the most obvious cases, before proceeding to notice those more delicate instances which are properly regarded as belonging to the Æsthetic class.

Painful feelings of considerable acuteness arise from exposure to any very powerful and persistent direct light. The sun, the voltaic arc, the calcium lamp, all rapidly fatigue the nerves of the eye. If the exposure is long continued, the feeling rises to a very painful pitch: and blindness results after a certain time, as in the barbaric torture of cutting off the eyelids. Even very short exposure yields a disagreeable dazzling sensation. Lights of lesser intensity, such as ordinary gas or kerosine lamps, fatigue the eyes if looked at directly for a few moments. Reflected light, when of moderate strength, similarly affects the nerves, as in the glare of sunshine from the water, or from mirrors, metal roofs, and shop windows. Even when far less intense, as in the case of wet pavements, snow-crystals, and dewy grass, the garish effect is highly disagreeable. Dispersed and scattered light is occasionally powerful enough sensibly to fatigue the sight. Soft snow, which does not directly reflect the sunshine, yet rapidly dazzles the eyes. In the tropics, white roads produce a like effect; and even in an English summer the glare of dusty streets is excessively unpleasant. Nor is it only the powerful stimulation of white light, affecting all three orders of fibres at once, that produces this result: red and orange in large quantities equally tire the special structures concerned; and the general diffused light of a very sunny day is decidedly disagreeable.

Besides these varieties of painful, because excessive, stimulation, there is another class of visual fatigues which is worth notice on account of its analogy to the case of dissonance. All intermittent and jerky stimulation of the optic nerve is unpleasant, because it attacks the fibres just as they are freshly repaired. To this class belong the unpleasant effects of flickering and unsteady lights, many of which have been already quoted. Gas and tallow candles, as well as fire-light, yield instances: while the mellow effect of daylight and moderator lamps is owing to their steadiness.

On the other hand, mere light is agreeable in proper quantities as stimulus after sleep and repose. In the night, if awake, we dislike the dark and long for morning. In the evening, we enjoy the lamp or gas, and object to gloomily-lighted rooms. Brilliant illumination is specially desired for dinner-parties, balls, and other festive occasions.* Savages seek similar pleasures in their torch-light dances. The light of day is agreeable, if not too strong. Sunshiny mornings are more pleasant than murky ones. As a relief from over-stimulation we insist upon the pleasure of a normal amount of light in a shady walk or a dim cathedral aisle. Poets and painters are fond of such subdued illumination, and dislike the garishness of full sunshine. In morbid states of nerve—as during headache—we require a darkened room. In

* Many readers may remember the ridiculous appearance of the London theatres during the gasmen's strike a few years since.

short, the due amount of action in the visual organ is pleasant. Gloom prevents us from fully carrying out our ordinary functions, and glare fatigues our eyes: but normal stimulation yields us a slight passive pleasure.

A more distinct kind of enjoyment is derived from separate points of light, when not too intense, in contrast to surrounding darkness, as in beacons, bonfires, illuminations, rockets, and catherine-wheels. The full moon, comets, and the stars yield similar pleasures. So do fire-flies, glow-worms, marine phosphorescence, and electrical phenomena. The aurora borealis exhibits the same effect on a grander scale. Even the lurid light which overhangs a great city, a house on fire, or an iron-smelting district, is not without a weird beauty of its own.

All these varieties of visual pleasure and pain depend entirely upon fatigue or normal stimulation of the optic nerve. But there is also another order of emotional phenomena connected with vision, depending rather upon the various muscles and contractile bodies which regulate the direction and convergence of the eyes, or the focussing of the organs for close or distant sight. If we try to fix our eyes steadily upon any single point for a long time, we are conscious of distinct muscular fatigue. If we dissociate the eyes, or gaze at any object too close for proper convergence, we feel a similar strain. In looking attentively at very small points, especially at a distance, we are easily tired. Rapidly revolving bodies weary us in the automatic attempt to follow their revolutions: if two adjacent ones revolve in opposite directions behind one another, the effect is positively painful. After a day's sight-seeing the eyes ache; and long continued reading produces a similar disagreeable feeling, sometimes accompanied by permanent disease. In fact, any excessive or exhausting demand upon the muscular apparatus of sight soon gives rise to more or less painful effects. It need hardly be added that as the muscles are very minute, the point of exhaustion is quickly reached. No very obvious instances of the corresponding pleasure can be cited; but this part of the subject will be more fully entered into when we come to examine beauty of form.

So far it will be noticed that we have merely considered the general pleasures and pains of total light, or of the muscular adjustments of sight, without any allusion to the special cases of form and colour. A few of the former, as in the case of fire-flies or the full moon, almost rise to the æsthetic level; but the greater part are the analogues of those emotional phenomena of sound which we regarded as outside the æsthetic class. We must now pass on to the more distinctively æsthetic visual manifestations.

§ 5. *Colour.*

Absolutely black and dull surfaces scatter no appreciable amount of light. All the rays which fall upon them are degraded to the form of heat. Consequently, they give no stimulation to the optic nerve. Hence blackness is always unpleasant, unless relieved by polish and consequent direct reflexion. A room hung with dull black is appalling in its sombreness. Black is the almost universal hue for mourning, and most of the fabrics used for the purpose are, like crape, as rough as possible. Here the original intention is to show sorrow by the complete absence of decorative colour. It takes a very pretty face to look well in widow's weeds. For a similar reason, black is used in the dress of nuns, where the object is to make the natural beauty of the features (if any) as unattractive as possible. When we employ black objects for decorative purposes, like jet, we give them the utmost attainable lustre; and we polish our boots after blacking them. At best, black in ordinary cases is emotionally neutral, and can only be made pleasurable by some super-added effect of reflexion, softness, or contrast; as in the ordinary combinations of black-and-gold, black-and-silver, or black-and-red.

White, on the other hand, though liable to become painful in an excessive light, is usually pleasing as a stimulant, but not so pungent as the analytic colours. Freshly fallen snow, spotless linen, white paper, are all more or less agreeable. Marble, either in statuary or architecture, is more decidedly æsthetic. White dresses, the Roman toga, or the modern bridal attire, have a certain simple beauty of their own. Probably these effects are chiefly due to the intensity of the scattered white light in each case, and its consequent power as an excitant. The whites of nature are mostly greyish in tinge: poets, on the contrary, dwell upon the purity and spotlessness of the white objects they introduce. The love for white in its full intensity gives rise to the processes of fulling and bleaching. A fleece on the sheep's back is a sorry-looking dirty tangle: when washed and combed into a hearth-rug it pleases us by its snowy hue as well as by its luxurious softness.

Between white and black, with little or no admixture of analytic colours, are innumerable shades of grey and mud-colour, which differ from pure white only in the ever-decreasing amount of rays which they reflect in proportion to those which they absorb. These are, on the whole, the least pleasing of all hues. They affect the nerves in the same manner as white, but with a slight and languid stimulation. Hence they have neither the pungency of red, green, and yellow, nor the purity of total white. They are very common in inorganic nature, and civilisation has brought them to the surface in our roads and streets. While green is the principal hue of the native fields, grey in various shades is the principal hue of the city.

Compared with the absolute negation of black, the familiar stimulation of white, and the duller excitement of the different greys, there is the pleasure of novelty and pungency in the strong irritation of the analytic colours, simple and compound—blue, green, yellow, orange, red, and purple. That these colours are in themselves pleasurable, especially when brilliant and pure, is undeniable. Not only do children and savages prize coloured objects, like feathers, beads, cloth, and pebbles, but the most refined taste is gratified by them in the rainbow, the hues of sunset, and the autumn tints upon the forest. The gratification is doubtless due to the powerful stimulation of the nerves in a special area by the single irritant. If the stimulation is excessive or protracted, pleasure soon yields to fatigue.

All these colours, however, are not equally pleasurable. In external nature, untouched by the hand of man, the violet end of the spectrum is much commoner than the red. On the hills and valleys around we see masses of green: in the clear sky above, an unbroken field of azure. But only an occasional flower, a stray butterfly, or a solitary bird yields us crimson, purple, or orange. From this arise several noticeable æsthetic results. In the first place, our eyes, having naturally adapted themselves to their circumstances, are capable of enduring much greater and more prolonged stimulation from green and blue surfaces than from red and yellow. Hence we prefer a preponderance of these hues in the visual field; we demand that a landscape should chiefly consist of sky and foliage; and we require abundant green as the background to a bouquet, which seems otherwise too staring. But on the other hand, the rarer stimulants of reds and yellows are more distinctly pleasurable in themselves, as arousing function in seldom-excited nerves; while the greens, blues, and greys are rather sought after as reliefs from excessive action. Furthermore, the colours of the red end would seem to have assigned to them weaker or less numerous fibres than those of the violet; which is only what we should expect from their lesser frequency. Accordingly they more rapidly fatigue the organs; and though admired in masses by coarse natures, children, and savages, they are only endurable by the refined in small amounts, properly relieved by other tints. Yet it will be immediately noticed that reds and other "warm" colours are much more frequent in artificial products, even the most refined, than in external nature; which clearly proves their pleasurable effect.

Indeed the very existence of reds, yellows, and purples in the outer world is indirectly almost entirely owing to their special effect upon animal organs. For though a few rare minerals, like the precious stones, exhibit brilliant colouring, and though many clays and sands show duller shades of these hues, yet for the most part they are found in the flowering parts of plants and in animal organisms. Now the flowers with brilliant corollas or stamens are those which are mainly fertilized by means of insects, and they generally have other allurements in the way of scent and honeyed secretions. Those on the other hand which are mainly fertilized by the wind are generally destitute of all these attractions. A moment's consideration will show us that a bright patch of colour in the midst of greens and greys would give a very pungent and special stimulation to a particular area in the eye. Hence those flowers which possessed such patches in the neighbourhood of their stamens and pistils would be readily discriminated by insects and birds. So, in the midst of the prevalent green of vegetable life, we find that patches of red, yellow, blue, and orange are developed around the floral organs of reproduction, as an aid to cross-fertilization. Night-flowering plants, on the other hand, have mostly large white blossoms which reflect all the possible light, thereby attracting the eyes of moths. Similarly with seeds. Those among them which bid for animal favour, like the pulpy sweet fruits, are rendered attractive not only by their taste and smell, but also by their brilliant hues, as in the orange, the mango, the cherry, and the plum. Hips and haws, holly-berries, and the bright scarlet capsicum are specially coloured to allure the eyes of birds. Conversely, those fruits which would be injured by animal interference, like the horse-chestnut and the filbert, are covered by a protective sheath of green when upon the tree, and brown when lying on the bare soil beneath. *Pari passu* with this development of brilliant colour in the vegetable world, must have come the development of a taste for brightness in the animal world. So that we have here another instance of the growth of that wider consensus between fauna and flora which we have already noticed in the case of taste and smell. The rise of this liking for visual pleasures aroused by unusual stimulants shows itself in the sexual selection of beautiful mates which has produced the crest of the newt, the plumage of the argus pheasant, the peacock, or the bird of paradise, and the brilliant hues of the baboon; not to mention the cherry lips, rosy cheeks, blue eyes, and golden hair of our Aryan maidens. Occasionally, too, the bright colouring serves rather to warn than to allure—like our own red danger-signals—as is the case with many insects whose tints are startlingly vivid, while their taste is disagreeable. Conversely, here again, as with the seeds and fruits, those insects which are liable to be preyed upon by birds or other enemies simulate closely the colouring of their environment.*

* This ground has already been sufficiently broken by Mr. Darwin, Professor Wallace, and Dr. Hooker; but they have rather pointed out the adaptation of these colours to the animal eye, while I wish more to insist upon the parallel adaptation of the eye to the colours. I had originally intended to

The distribution of colours in the environment which is thus partial has produced a like partial distribution of colour-perceiving elements in the retina. Many facts concur to prove that there are fewer fibres for the perception of red than for the perception of any other colour; and that these fibres require a stronger stimulant to produce sensation than is the case with any others. The peripheral portions of the retina are incapable of perceiving red; and white, when seen on these portions assumes a complementary greenish tint.* If we try to perceive very small or imperfectly illuminated figures, those coloured red are the least easily perceived of any. And in a common abnormality, known as colour-blindness (or more correctly, *dichroism*), the power of perceiving the red rays, alone or in composition, is wholly wanting. All these facts point alike to a comparative weakness and scarcity of the red-perceiving elements. And a moment's consideration will show us that this is just the effect which we might expect to see produced by natural selection. For it is clearly desirable that the eyes of the frugivorous animals should be pleasurably stimulated by reds, oranges, and purples; and the simplest contrivance for effecting this end would be to give the greatest possible rest to such elements as answer to stimulations of these orders. Accordingly, they ought to be only excited by comparatively powerful stimulations of their proper kind. How greatly habits of life may alter the conformation of the eye can be

follow out this subject in a chapter on "The Genesis of Æsthetics," but have decided not to do so for want of space.

* See the next section.

seen by considering the case of nocturnal animals, whose retina shows peculiarities which probably indicate an absence of the mechanism for the perception of separate colours, and a presence of that for the discrimination of light in varying intensity alone.

We may conclude accordingly that patches of bright colour, especially red, yellow, and purple, always attract the unsophisticated eye, in the midst of prevalent greys, browns, and greens. Children delight in gathering handfuls of way-side flowers, though they have not skill enough to relieve them by interspersing sufficient foliage. But flowers quickly die, and grown savages are not content with such transitory possessions. Hence the value attached to any bright-coloured object which permanently retains its tints. While roses and peonies, starfish and sea-anemonies, soon fade away and become positively unpleasant, shells, feathers, pebbles, pearls, and seeds are prized as personal decorations. The precious metals delight the savage eye by their glitter; and it is a curious thought that the commerce of the civilized world is still carried on by bartering the shining baubles which once hung round the necks of barbarian chiefs. Soon the discovery of pigments is made: the bow or the basket is stained yellow, blue, or red. To this stage belong the purple-dyed ivory and the gold-studded sceptre. Bits of cloth are stained for personal attire, the brightest hues being preferred. Colour becomes an attribute of state and royalty; the simple throne, the kingly dress, and the royal hut are conspicuous for their gorgeous tints. At last we get the application of colour to imitative purposes, and art proper begins. This final stage must be considered in a later chapter.

We must remember that in all such questions as these concerning the intrinsic beauty of colours we should always take as our standard the simple sense of savages, children, and uneducated adults. In our own time men of culture, revolted by the preference vulgarly given to strong stimulants, prefer the more delicate tints, neutral colours, and pale or subdued primaries, to the staring dyes which they see around them. But with primitive man the case is different. Red and purple are to him novelties, and his coarser organisation is not easily fatigued by their effects. Even in modern houses furnished with the most fastidious taste as to wall-paper and dado, carved oak and dainty coverings, it will be found that reds and yellows are far more conspicuous than in external nature. Nobody has yet succeeded in expelling them from his conservatory.

Under the present heading we may interpolate the pleasure derived from lustre; that is, from the reflected light of polished surfaces. This pleasure is partly intellectual, and consists in a recognition of tactual smoothness in the lustrous object; but it is also in part immediate, and is derived from the acute stimulation of total light. By means of lustre, blackness can be considerably relieved, and may even become an agreeable rest for the nerves by the side of the bright surface. Lustre also adds an extra beauty to white and to the brilliant analytic colours. In leaves and flowers this effect is generally obtained by immediate reflexion from the transparent cell-walls; while the coloured light is scattered by the more deeply-seated pigment matter. It is constantly imitated by art, as in the varnish on oil-paintings and furniture, or the polish on statuettes and porcelain-ware. Conversely with dullness: not only is there an unpleasant suggestion of gritty touch, but also we miss the agreeable stimulation of immediately reflected light. Hence the invention of varnish, lacquer, and all the other expedients by which we glaze over or smoothen the surface of rough and dull objects. But in all these cases the visual and tactual elements, in the actuality and in the idea, are so closely bound up with one another, and with complex emotional feelings, that a complete separation even in mental analysis is almost impossible.

For example, white by its physical purity suggests the poetical analogy of moral purity, and this again re-acts upon our sense of white. Hence we see a peculiar propriety in white as the garb of the virgin bride, of the first communion, and of religious service; and we further extend its use to angels and other ideally pure beings. On the other hand, black by its dullness and gloom is appropriated to purposes of mourning; and this idea, too, re-acts so as to give us an associated distaste for black, which we further picture as the complexion of devils, goblins, and evil spirits. But when once black has come to have a conventional association with death, we may for purposes of state and show so mitigate its unpleasantness by considerations of form and costliness as to leave merely a sense of solemn magnificence. Such mitigation is attempted in a ceremonial funeral, with its sable horses, crape drapery, black waving plumes, and polished hearse.

Though the pleasures here considered are not of a very high type, being so little discriminative and so universal, yet they undoubtedly belong to the lower stratum of Æsthetic Feelings. Those which we have next to examine claim a higher rank.

§ 6. *Harmony and Discord of Colour.*

We have seen in the last section that certain masses of colour are in themselves, apart from any effects of combination, pleasurable stimulants of the optic nerve. They may thus be regarded as the analogues of musical tones, which we saw to be similarly gratifying in isolation, because they aroused normal amounts of action in fully-nurtured and under-worked nervous structures. But most pleasures of colour are not so simple in their nature as these, nor do those we have already considered rank very high in æsthetic value. Savages are pleased by yards of red or blue cloth, and even cultured eyes are often attracted by a colour of unusual purity and richness, unrelieved by contrast or harmony: but the greater number of artistic effects depend upon combinational considerations. We found in Hearing that the peculiar fact upon which consonance and dissonance were based was that of interference, and the consequent production of beats; we have now to enquire what is the corresponding physical fact upon which is founded the feeling of harmony and discord in the perception of colour.

We have seen already, that if we gaze for a moderate time

upon the sun or an incandescent object like the carbon-points of a voltaic arc, our optic nerve is rapidly fatigued. If we then look away at any uniformly illuminated surface, such as the white-washed ceiling, we are conscious of a dark patch, having the same shape as the object with which we have tired our eyes. This dark patch does not remain stationary, but follows the motion of the eyes. The reason for this phenomenon is as follows. The direct light from the incandescent body fell upon a certain area in the retina; all the nerves having their terminations in that area are consequently quite exhausted, and can yield us little or no sensation until they have undergone a comparatively lengthy repair. But the surrounding area is still fresh and unexhausted; and accordingly all parts of the retina except this wearied patch perform their functions correctly. Such patches of wearied nerves give rise to sensations known as *negative accidental images*, to distinguish them from another class called *positive*, of no great importance to our present question.

The negative image which we have just considered was produced by total light falling upon the retina. But cases also occur where æther-waves of a particular frequency alone, giving rise to a sensation of analytic colour, fatigue certain portions of the retina, and are followed by a negative image of a different colour. For example, if we gaze steadily for a few minutes at a bright green figure, and then withdraw the eyes and fix them upon the ceiling, we shall see a corresponding figure, subtending an equal angle, and apparently coloured pale red. The reason of this is analogous to the previous case. The green rays have fatigued the green-perceiving fibres of the optic nerve, terminating in that portion of the retina, and they no longer yield their full amount of sensation. But the other fibres of the same area are unaffected by the green rays, and consequently retain all their freshness. So, while the green rays reflected from the ceiling in the total light produce no effect, the remaining rays, in which red preponderates, arouse action in their corresponding nerves and terminal organs, and the sensation is cognised as faint red. Similarly, a red object is followed by a green image, and a blue object by a yellow one. In short, whenever one set of nervous structures is fatigued, a negative image appears, and is seen of a certain other colour which, when combined with the original incident colour, produces the sensation of whiteness. Colours which when so combined yield white light are said to be complementary.

These facts have been introduced because they give the best proof of the general principle that light of any particular colour falling upon the eye fatigues those nerves only which answer to it as a stimulant. In this partial exhaustion we get the ground-work for the pleasures and pains of harmonious and discordant colouring. In the cases already quoted, the fatigue of the eyes can be distinctly recognised as such, and hence they fail to come up to the æsthetic level of mere intellectual perception. After practical experiments in seeing negative images, the eyes ache. But when we recognise a discord between two adjacent colours, we do not set down our dislike to conscious fatigue; we know the effect only as an æsthetic feeling. Hence these cases are strictly analogous to the instance of hearing. Recurrent interferences up to a certain point of frequency are cognized as beats: beyond it, we saw that they were only known as dissonance.

It may, however, be objected that this principle of fatigue could only apply to successive, not to simultaneous and adjacent colours. Such is actually the fact. Our eyes are perpetually moving in a restless manner from point to point in the field of vision, even when we are not aware of it; and only a very small area in that field can be distinctly cognised at one and the same instant. Hence the portions of the retina affected by adjacent regions of the visual field are in a constant state of interchange. Accordingly, if we have in one place a patch of red, the portion of the retina which is receiving light from it will have its red-perceiving fibres strongly excited and, as a necessary consequence, fatigued. If, next, it is directed upon a neighbouring patch of green, the red-perceiving fibres will be at rest, and undergo repair, while the fresh and vigorous green-perceiving structures will receive normal stimulation. Hence such interchange of colours will be pleasurable. But if, on the contrary, it is immediately directed upon a patch of purple or orange, which will make fresh demands upon the wearied red-perceiving fibres, the effect will be that disagreeable feeling which we call a discord. So that all colour-harmony consists in such an arrangement of tints as will give the various portions of the retina stimulation in the least fatiguing order, and all colour-discord in the opposite.*

* I learn from milliners and dress-makers that after sewing for a long time

Actual experience shows us that such is the case. The famous colour-harmony of the Italian painters, red, green, and violet, is that which rouses action successively in all three classes of fibres, so that the eye can range freely over the whole field of combination without exhaustion, and with ever-refreshed enjoyment, thus yielding, in accordance with our formula, the maximum of stimulation with the minimum of fatigue.* Blue and bright yellow, purple and green, violet and orange, form similar tasteful combinations; while green and blue, green and yellow, orange and red, yield most unpleasant results. In each case it will be noticed that those combinations give pleasure which call into play the most different fibres; while those produce discord which successively stimulate the same class of structures.

Here, too, we see the reason for the occasional relative pleasurableness of black. By itself it is disagreeable or neutral, but when combined with certain varieties of light it becomes negatively pleasant: that is to say, it gives the eye time for repair in the intervals of stimulation. Hence the favourite colours for combination with black are those which most rapidly fatigue the nerves, so redressing the balance. Gold or silver are in themselves too pungent; the excessive gilding of mirrors and picture frames is an infallible token of bad taste. But when sparingly employed on a background

upon discordant materials, such as they occasionally have to make up, their eyes distinctly ache. I may add that they are unusually discriminative of this class of feelings.

* It is due to Professor Bain to state that this formula was originally (though unconsciously) adopted by me from a chance expression of his in dealing with colour-harmony alone. I did not discover my obligation to him for the phrase till the earlier parts of this work were ready for publication.

of black, they become mild enough for the most fastidious eye. We have seen already that red is a specially fatiguing colour; and its various shades go well with black both in dress and art. Green, blue, and violet, on the contrary, are not pungent enough to stand this relief. Negresses look best in scarlet or yellow turbans, which add colour to their otherwise neutral faces: blues and greens do not suit them. The black and crimson Canadian soldier-bird is one of the loveliest natural objects I have ever seen. In the case of polished black surfaces we get side by side brilliant patches of light and total darkness. In short, the real pleasure in every instance is derived from the positive light, and the blackness only acts as a repairer or non-stimulant; but we imagine it to be pleasurable by a parallel illusion to that which leads us to consider it as a colour instead of a mere negation. Strip off the red bows, or the gold and silver trimmings, and what becomes of a black dress?

Similarly with other combinations. In arranging flowers, we need a copious interspersed background of green. Take a piece of holly with the berries attached, and nothing can be prettier than the effect of the dark verdure and the brilliant scarlet: pull off all the leaves, and the berries remain a mere staring mass of red. Foliage does not show off well as it grows: but we can better admire the delicate green of a fern if we hold it against a field of dark brown. Again, much depends upon the effect which we wish to produce. Green and gold form a bright and beautiful mixture; purple and grey have a more solemn and severe appearance; white needs relief with black or dark blue; while red requires bright green for liveliness, and darker tints for subdued harmony. Moreover, masses of colour which, if taken by themselves and at close quarters, fatigue the eyes, are pleasant at a short distance, when they only form a single element in the visual field. Thus the dress of a soldier is by itself hideously over-stimulating; taken as one element of a landscape it is effective. Painters put old women in red cloaks as a warm foreground to their pieces. But such colours taken in large quantities are unendurable. In an ordinary ball room, the black coats of the men serve as a foil for the white, pink, and light blue dresses of the women. At a regimental, Masonic, or Highland dance, the varied mass of unrelieved colour, heightened by the glare of gas, has a somewhat barbaric extravagance. In a Gothic cathedral, the crimson light from the painted windows is toned down by the solemn grey of the walls : a Byzantine church gives us gold and scarlet till the stimulation is overwhelming in its intensity. Great taste in the selection and blending of colours may somewhat diminish the unpleasant effect, as in the empirically-obtained harmonies of Moorish decoration (which mainly depend upon the smallness of each separate coloured area, so that the eye can wander rapidly from one to the other) : but even while we allow the highest praise to the skill exhibited, we feel that the æsthetic effect is produced rather by well-sustained pungency than by more delicate interventions of relieving tints.*

It will be unnecessary to add further examples. Starting

* The amount of each colour—primary, secondary, or tertiary—needed to balance the total effect is given in Field's scale of Chromatic Equivalents.

from these simple cases, it is easy to see that we may progress to every possible combination, only requiring for their perception more and more discriminative nervous organizations. It will also be obvious that the pleasures and pains of harmony and discord are far higher in the æsthetic scale than those of the simple colours: so much so that they almost escape children and savages, and are only fully appreciated by the most delicate organs. We may leave these and similar questions to be filled in by the experience of the reader, and pass on to the second great division of visual sensations.

§ 7. *Form.*

Colour, we have seen, depends upon the class of optical nerve-fibres differentially affected: Form depends upon their number and relative position.

This remark, however, must be accepted in the strictest sense as applicable to visible form alone.

The eye has originally only two modes of perception, that of colour and that of plane figure. Distance is recognised by certain combinations of these and the muscular adjustment of the organ; and form in three dimensions is a compound of colour in the way of shading with plane figure. All questions respecting these belong entirely to the intellectual half of our nature; beauty of Form is chiefly concerned with the muscular sweep of the eye in cognizing adjacent points.

We saw above that when the muscles or contractile bodies of the eye are employed for any length of time in observing a single point or in following rapid and perplexing movements, fatigue supervenes. Now the painful effect of all unpleasant forms is due to a modified and very slight exhaustion of a similar kind. Conversely, the agreeable feeling derived from all graceful forms is due to the easy and unimpeded action of the muscles and other tissues concerned. These cases, however, are so very minute in their nature as almost to defy regular analysis, and it will accordingly be necessary to approach them in a somewhat different manner from that which we have usually adopted.

Straight lines are almost, if not quite, unknown in nature. Whenever we see a straight row of trees or plants, we know that they have been sown by the hand of man; whenever we come upon a straight stream of water, we recognize it as a canal of human construction. But in the woods and the rivers, all is careless and unconstrained. As soon as the human race begins to use its hands for constructive purposes, the straight line is recognised as the most convenient boundary for many objects. In building, it commends itself as being the most stable form; in weapons, as being the most unerring. Moreover, it has a regularity and perfection which naturally contrasts with the uneven handiwork of nature. So the straight line comes gradually to be employed for a vast number of purposes, until at last its infrequency in the savage world is almost forgotten. In the rooms where we live we find the walls and the ceiling straight; the tables and cupboards, the doors and windows, are bounded by straight lines; the very panes and panels, the lock and the hearth-rug, are all rectangular. This page is cut to an even edge, and all the letters are arranged in regular rows. In every one of these facts, and in a dozen more which a single glance around him will reveal to the reader, we see that love of order and symmetry which is so deeply seated in civilized man, and whose origin must form the subject-matter of a succeeding section. We must accordingly allow a certain æsthetic value—intellectual rather than sensuous—to the straight line; which none can doubt except that class of mystical thinkers who consider merely the most complex artistic developments instead of beginning with the simplest elements. Even those who most strenuously deny the beauty of the straight line would hardly give any other limiting boundary to a picture, a book, or a room.

If, however, we follow up with our sight a straight line which proceeds for some distance, we shall find that a distinctly awkward motion of the head and eyes is necessary for its perception. Still more clearly can we notice that the attempt to take in any rectangular figure involves a considerable expenditure of muscular energy. Figures with very acute or re-entrant angles are yet more trying. And as soon as we really direct our attention to the subject, we find that we can only observe a very small figure at a time without re-adjustment of the visual organs. In observing angular shapes this re-adjustment is required for every angle. A curve, on the contrary, being coincident with the natural sweep of the organs, is easily and carelessly perceived. A series of curves, like Hogarth's line of grace, can be followed without difficulty. An excellent opportunity for trying the experiment may often be found in the comparison of a modern rectangular casement of church-warden architecture with the flowing tracery of an adjacent flamboyant window. The first symptom of nascent architectural taste in English villas and cottages may be traced in the introduction of an arched door-way, a rounded alcove, or a bow window. In this faint emotional difference we have the simplest origin for the distinction of graceful and awkward forms.

The necessity for variety gives us another supplementary basis, more purely optical, but largely mixed with intellectual elements. Sameness in outline will demand continuous exertion of the same muscles, combined with continued stimulation of the same retinal points. Variety in figure implies variety in stimulation. Hence, in part, the pleasure which we feel in looking over a field of vision full of varied and novel forms and colours; as well as the converse discomfort of flatness, monotony, and uniformity in shape and hue.

Again, the eyes are specially restless organs, not only laterally and vertically, but also in their focus for nearer and further distances. When we are obliged to keep our eyes fixed for a considerable period upon a single point, as in having our photographs taken, the effort is extremely fatiguing. So too a look-out from a window upon a straight flat wall, besides its intellectual meagreness, tires us by the uniformity of focus which it demands. Hence in architecture a façade on a single plane is very wearisome: we require porticos, arches, projecting turrets, and other salient points, which attract the eyes and keep them wandering over the whole elevation with constant grateful changes of focus and muscular sweep. And in a landscape we admire hills which lie one behind another in perspective; vistas through avenues or interlacing boughs; large objects in the foreground breaking up the monotony of the focal distance; and a background of decided objects, upon which the eye can rest with that arrangement for long vision which makes the least call upon the muscles regulating the shape of the crystalline lens.

Lastly, a portion of the pleasure usually assigned to this heading is not really due to true perceptions of Form, but to the pleasing variety of colour which is given by shading, relief, and perspective.

I am aware that the explanation thus vaguely sketched is a very imperfect one, far less immediately physical than those which have hitherto been given; but for this imperfection two excuses can be pleaded: in the first place, the pleasure of Form is far higher and more delicate than that of colour, and far less amenable to fixed rules—which is equivalent to saying that its emotional factors are far more minute and inscrutable; while, in the second place, so involuted and interdependent are the various elements of Æsthetic Feelings, that we cannot examine the intellectual till we have catalogued the sensuous, and yet cannot explain the sensuous without the aid of the intellectual. Though colours are often beautiful in utter isolation, (as in the clear blue of a cloudless sky, or the delicate crimson of vinegar in which beet-root has been steeped,) hardly any single line can be said to possess beauty of itself, apart from intellectual considerations of symmetry and proportion. To these, then, we next proceed.*

§ 8. *Symmetry.*

The pleasures and pains we have hitherto examined are those of normal or excessive stimulation in the optic nerve, and those of due exercise or fatigue in the various motor appliances of the eye. We have now to notice a species of emotional feelings which are connected with the higher perceptive centres, and are commonly described as intellectual. They will form the subject of the succeeding chapter, but a few remarks concerning them must be interpolated here, in order to complete our view of the visual Æsthetic Feelings.

Observations made on persons with congenital cataract, afterwards couched, have shown that for some time after gaining the faculty of vision they are troubled and distressed by the vast mass of shifting visual sensations perpetually poured in upon them. The intellect is unable to co-ordinate these various perceptions so as to draw from them any reasonable impression. It is only by slow degrees that their relations to the various tactual counterparts are perceived: and meanwhile the effect produced is one of mere

* In this section I have only endeavoured to work out the purely sensuous or presentative elements of beauty in form: the reader will find the ideal or representative elements fully considered in Mr. Herbert Spencer's Essay on *Gracefulness.* The exact nature of those curves and sections which yield pleasurable feelings is fully considered by the late Dr. Symonds in his *Miscellanies,* and still more lately by Fechner in his *Vorschule der Æsthetik.*

bewilderment. This necessarily involves waste of nervous energy, for it implies unsuccessful efforts at co-ordination. In an infant we have some signs of the same bewilderment, but it is not so obviously displayed, because the higher co-ordinating centres are still in a very undeveloped state, and the corresponding tactual sensations are as unknown as the visual forms by which they are symbolized. The period at which an infant begins to correlate sights with touches and tastes is marked by very apparent symptoms, technically known to nurses as "taking notice." After this period, changes in the visible surroundings are rapidly observed, and the obtrusion of unknown objects is followed by fear or perplexity. These feelings give way in the child to shyness, and in the adult to a more or less languid curiosity. But even at a mature age something of the youthful consternation is revived on the first visit to a great city, a foreign country, or a society to which we are unused. In all, we experience an unpleasant bewilderment, a difficulty in ordering our conduct so as to meet the requirements of the untried situation.

On the other hand, we are always pleased at any such familiar arrangement as at once enables us to frame our action aright. After a few weeks abroad, the look of English streets, the habits of English hotels, the dress of English policemen, all assure us that we have returned to comparatively well-known surroundings. A map or plan of a city enables us to reduce its chaos of streets to a mental order. Country walks are rendered far more interesting if we know the various surrounding landmarks, and can identify hill or cape, seen from different points of view. In short, everywhere that which suggests the idea of knowledge and comprehensibility is pleasing: that which wastes the energy of the higher nervous organs in useless conjecture is disagreeable.

Now I will not affirm that our love of symmetry and order is immediately dependent upon such considerations, or that it owes nothing to other utilitarian sources; but I believe that it is closely cognate with these intellectual feelings. A mere tangled mass of sensations, without order or plan, strikes us as meaningless or absolutely disagreeable: a regular arrangement of parts yields us a mental gratification in following out its various portions, and recognizing its apparent design. But while the emotional feelings described above are not regarded as æsthetic, because they are connected with the due regulation of our practical conduct, the feelings aroused by orderly or disorderly arrangement of parts, being unconnected with such useful ends, are elevated into the æsthetic rank. We have been taught in our observation of organic bodies to expect regularity, and we imitate it ourselves in art. A few cases of each will suffice.

The leaves of plants for the most part exhibit a symmetrical arrangement on either side of the midrib. Leaves like those of ferns, which show the symmetrical order both in the whole and in its various parts, with considerable variety of contour, are the most admired. Others in which symmetry is slightly marked and variety wanting, like burdock or cabbage, have small claims to beauty. Those flowers which bid for animal observation by their scents, secretions, and brilliant colours, are also noticeable for the systematic order of the corolla and its adjuncts. Many have the petals arranged in a radial form, and their edges rounded or pinked. Others have their various colours symmetrically disposed, like the daisy, the fuchsia, and the tiger-lily. If we proceed to the animal world we see, in the lower grades of life, the radiated or circular arrangement of star-fish, sea-anemones, and echini, all of which are beautiful objects. Above them come the double shells of bivalve mollusca, and the regular spirals of univalves. Amongst the articulata and vertebrata, symmetry is usually bilateral, but still very noticeable, alike in the butterfly and the beetle, the swan and the deer. On the other hand, all apparently amorphous creatures, like the oyster, the slug, and the polypus, besides all species which depart from the usual bilateral symmetry, as is the case with soles and flounders, strike us with a certain disgust. Even abnormal distribution of colour, as in piebald horses or port-wine stains, is by no means so pretty as the regular speckling of trout and guinea-fowl. Everywhere, regularity pleases us, and disorder repels or at least fails to attract.

From the constant sight of all these symmetrical objects and others like them, and from the contemplation of his own fellows, primeval man learns to expect a regular order of parts under certain circumstances.* Most of the above instances occur in perishable objects; but, as in the case of colour,

* On the connection between symmetry in animal forms and in Greek architecture, see Mr. Herbert Spencer's Essay on the *Sources of Architectura Types.*

whenever symmetry is found in any permanent natural products, like shells, corals, seeds, and crystals, they are prized as personal decorations. When he begins to combine coloured feathers or pebbles for his own adornment, he arranges them in recurring orders. As soon as he has learnt the use of pigments, he paints his bow in equal strips of alternate red, green, and yellow. His calabash and his earthen pot are decorated with circles and crosses at measured distances. His own person is tattooed in curves and figures. In his earliest attempts at weapons he gives his stone hatchet and his arrow-head a rough symmetry, which in remains of the neolithic period has developed into considerable artistic finish. The dances and processions in which the savage delights are arranged circularly or in even rank and file. His first lessons in architecture consist in rings, like Stonehenge, avenues, like Carnac, or regular rounded tumuli. When, with advancing culture, he begins to imitate nature in stone or colours, every object is perfectly symmetrical. All the men have two sides exactly alike; all the trees consist of branches at equal distances; and all the flowers grow at regular intervals. We get numerous instances of such symmetrical art in the Egyptian and Assyrian remains. Children draw after the same fashion to the present day. Later on we get symmetrical figures on textile fabrics and pottery, the well-known Greek key-pattern, arabesques, and the geometrical designs of wall-papers, carpets, and encaustic tiles. To illustrate once more by the room in which my reader is sitting, the table-cover, the anti-macassars, and the centre-piece of the ceiling, consist of circular ornaments, radially arranged; the globes of the glass chandelier have a regular pattern, and its branches are at equal angles: there is a conventional design on the banner-screen, and even the holes in the fire-shovel form an orderly figure. In higher walks of art, the columns of a Corinthian temple have fixed intervals; they are regularly arranged into corresponding parts; and their capitals are symmetrically carved. The tracery of a rose-window forms a geometrical pattern, and so do those of the perpendicular lights. Indeed, architecture generally is eminently characterized by symmetry, especially in all points of detail: and the same is even more strikingly the case with the art of internal decoration. Geometrical designs and conventional figures are now almost universally adopted for this purpose.

All that is here asserted about symmetry will doubtless meet with strenuous denial from a certain class of transcendental art-critics, who think that highest style of art alone worthy of analysis which satisfies their highly cultivated taste. They are fond of asserting, on the contrary, that there is *no* beauty in symmetry, and that real art is always unsymmetrical. The answer lies in an appeal to facts. That symmetry is pleasing to the vast majority of minds is conclusively shown by its almost universal employment in every form of decoration, from flower-gardens to crotchet-work. On the other hand, in those arts which aim at the imitation of nature it is obviously out of place, because symmetry in nature holds only a subordinate position. Each leaf and each flower is regularly arranged, but in the tree and the landscape, as they strike the eye, hardly a trace of regularity can be seen. Hence imitative art soon outgrows the trammels of conventional arrangement. Even in architectural and decorative art an occasional breach of symmetry is beautiful by contrast as a novelty. But it is only the general employment of symmetry that makes its absence a pleasing variety. A building in which every door, every window, every arch, and every pinnacle was placed irregularly would strike us as a mere chaotic monstrosity. Irregular (though bilateral) flowers, like the orchis and the snap-dragon, or unsymmetrical leaves, like the begonia, please us only by their singularity, as interesting though concordant divergences from an ordinary type. But in making bouquets we always reject broken or imperfect leaves, and flowers some of whose petals have been blighted or cramped. An educated taste admires variety, but all alike are revolted by obvious disorder and anarchic confusion.

It need only be added that symmetrical figures, like all others, must bow to the general laws both of form and colour. Straight lines and angles must be avoided; graceful and flowing curves must be introduced; and harmony must be carefully studied. Circular forms are most in favour for geometrical patterns. When all these requirements are fulfilled, as in the best internal ecclesiastical decoration, symmetrically arranged figures, though falling far short of imitative art, may and do excite comparatively high forms of æsthetic pleasure.*

* On the whole of this subject the reader may consult with advantage Mr. Owen Jones's *Grammar of Ornament*, which is written in a philosophic spirit rarely found in æsthetic works.

§ 9. *Concrete Æsthetic Objects owing their Beauty to Visual Qualities.*

Before we pass on to the imitative arts, it will be necessary to enter briefly into the question of intellectual and ideal feelings, which hold such an important position in Poetry, Painting, and Sculpture. These will appropriately form the subject of two separate chapters. But it may be well, after so long an exposition, to give a few concrete instances of objects in external nature, or in simple human products, which derive their beauty from colour, form, or symmetry, in various combinations.

Colour and bright light alone give beauty to the sunset: a faint element of regularity and curved form is added in the rainbow. Iridescence pleases us by its rapid interchange of hues: it is illustrated in the soap-bubble for a moment; in mother-of-pearl and the opal more permanently. Certain glazed porcelains and Venetian glass imitate artificially the same effect. Plants have beauty of form with bright green colouring. Their leaves have usually variety and symmetry. Fern, maple, parsley, and horse-chestnut leaves depend mainly upon these elements. Arum, holly, laurel, hart's-tongue, and the young leaves of ivy are beautiful for their brilliant green and glossiness. The foliage of the vine owes much to its exquisite venation. Those leaves which are both dull and shapeless are emotionally neutral or positively ugly. Among trees, the palms have drooping feathery branches; the conifers, tapering forms and symmetrical boughs; the weeping willow, graceful curves. Flowers need no special illustration. Shells, besides their brilliant tints, have curved or spiral forms, and many, like pecten and scalaria, are fluted or crenated. Some have coloured bands regularly arranged; others exhibit in their lips the most dainty pink or violet. A few are delicately transparent; they taper to the finest point, and astonish us by the minuteness and elegance of their workmanship: these depend for effect mainly upon form, symmetry, and variety. Oyster-shells, on the contrary, are both dull and shapeless. Butterflies have lovely colours and graceful forms: they flit easily from flower to flower, and chase one another in rhythmical curves. Some add lustre to their other attractions, while many are remarkable for the extraordinary purity and marvellous shading of their hues. Several beetles are burnished like gold, though their forms are ungainly and heavy. But birds bear away the palm of beauty from all competitors—indeed, their highly-developed æsthetic tastes are shown alike in their form, their colour, and their song. The bird-of-paradise has an exquisite shape, soft and plumy feathers, marvellous harmony and delicacy of colour, and perfect symmetry combined with freedom from stiffness. The last-named charge may perhaps be urged against the lyre-bird, which is faultless in all other respects. The peacock and the argus-pheasant at once occur to the readers of Mr. Darwin. The humming-birds have every beauty under heaven, except song: the amethyst, ruby, and sapphire of their throats are absolutely unsurpassed in art or nature. Even the less showy birds, like the heron, the swan, and the plover, show exquisite varieties of form. The dove has delicate colour and a graceful shape. The very crows and magpies are beautiful after their kind. Indeed there is scarcly such a thing as an ugly bird, if we except some species of owls, vultures and turkey-buzzards. Mammals are as a rule less beautiful, especially in colour. Those which please us in this respect are more remarkable for their delicate greys or browns than for brilliancy of analytic hues, as in the case of antelopes, pumas, quaggas, and hares. Others are striped, like the zebra and the tiger, or spotted like the fallow-deer and the giraffe. All these have beauty of form as well. Stags have slender legs and branching antlers; gazelles, a graceful body and tender eye; while the various larger cats are noticeable for their ease of movement and the gliding motion of their limbs beneath the skin. Bears, rhinoceroses and hippopotami, on the contrary, are dull, shapeless, and heavy. Lastly, man and woman unite all the beauties of form and colour, symmetry and variety, with every kind of complex emotional interest.

If we pass on from these separate elements to the greater totals which form natural scenery, we shall see (omitting for the present ideal factors) that all the varieties of visual pleasure enter into its composition, together with many intellectual gratifications. We have brilliant colouring in green fields, blue sky, purple sea, and cliffs of red marl or white chalk. Relief is present, if necessary, in the mild stimulation of black ploughed fields, grey cloud, or bare and craggy mountain-top. The snowy summits of the Alps shine with dazzling whiteness, and the fleecy clouds are tinged with gold or silver. Curved form is found in sweeping bay, and winding stream, and undulating down, and sloping hillside. Variety is given us in all the prospect. Flat and monotonous fields fatigue us. The desert, with its hot level expanse of grey sand, sweltering and blinking in the full glare of a tropical sun, is our ideal of utter dullness.* The unbroken green of western prairies is scarcely less tiring. The sea without a sail, as seen from mid-ocean, is miserably dull: a whale, a porpoise, or even a good foaming gale, is hailed as a grateful variety. When in search of æsthetic pleasure, we seek the interchange of hill and dale, river and waterfall, castle and abbey, green valley and ice-clad height. We climb downs for the extended view, spend our holiday at the sea-side for the sake of cliffs and water, or ransack Iceland, Ceylon, and Colorado in search of picturesque novelty in geyser and volcano, palm and tree-fern, cañon and lava-plain. Symmetry alone we reject, because we have learnt to associate that with the puny works of man, or when we find it in the outer world to expect it only in detail. Our notions of sublimity require that in her grandest achievements Nature should not be tied down to rule and plummet.

The same considerations apply to dress, textile fabrics, pottery, and other human products; but here, on the contrary, symmetry is imperatively demanded. Vases have usually beauty of curved form, applicability to their special function, colour either in a single delicate retiring shade, or else in harmonious combination, and symmetrical arrangement of parts. The loveliest fictile objects give us a double

* I am reminded by a friend that painters are rather fond of a caravan in the desert. That is true, because the monotonous sky-line brings out the camels in strong statuesque relief. But nobody ever dreamt of painting the desert without the camels.

curve, horizontal and perpendicular, thus yielding the maximum beauty of simple form. Glass is sometimes coloured, but more often depends on form alone, with the accompaniment of a regular pattern in a rougher ground surface. Dress is systematically arranged to be graceful in shape, harmonious in colour, and adapted to the individual who wears it. The ballet perhaps exhibits it in perfection. Internal decorations, as already noticed, are usually in geometrical figures. Colour enters largely into their effect. Architecture depends almost entirely upon form: it exhibits the sweeping arch, Romanesque or Gothic, the vaulted dome, and the interlacing branches of the painted window. Symmetry here is all important. Variety, too, counts for much. But, above all, intellectual appreciation is a prime factor in the æsthetic pleasure of architecture.

These human additions go far to enliven natural beauty. The unrelieved vegetation of tropical mountain scenery yields us the painful consciousness of an emotional blank. We long for the sight of man's handiwork. All must have been struck in Scottish lochs or Alpine passes with the unexpected pleasure when a turn in our course suddenly reveals some ruined fortress perched upon the crag, or mouldering abbey nestling in the vale. Sion, Fribourg, and Chillon form as important factors in our memories of Switzerland as do Pfäffers, the Giesbach, and the Mer-de-glace. Those who have compared the Rhine and the Hudson, the latter of which possesses every natural superiority and is disfigured by every architectural monstrosity, can appreciate Mr. Ruskin's objection to visit a country which has no castles. Even far less imposing structures have a beauty of their own. The light-house at the Needles, the Swiss châlet on the mountain-side, the Terrapin Tower at Niagara, each add to the effect of their several scenes. It is interesting, too, to compare the amount of æsthetic value to be attributed in each case to nature and to art. Hill and bay have done everything for Torquay, and man has done his best to spoil them. The lagoon of Venice is a mere stagnant pool, but it has been made lovely by the noblest architecture in Europe. Edinburgh, Naples, and Athens owe an equal debt to natural and artificial beauty.

With this necessarily brief list of a few leading visual æsthetic objects we may proceed to our analysis of the intellectual and ideal feelings, which form a large element of artistic enjoyment.

CHAPTER VIII.

THE INTERVENTION OF THE INTELLECT.

§ 1. *General Emotional Phenomena of the Intellect.*

THE pleasures and pains which we have hitherto considered are those aroused by normal or excessive function in the peripheral end-organs of nerves, or in the fibres and central end-organs immediately connected with them. But there is a higher class of nervous structures in the human system, whose business it is to correlate and co-ordinate the energies so received, and, where necessary, to liberate—immediately or ultimately—in accordance with the intelligence conveyed by these impressions, new energies which re-act upon the external world in the manner demanded by the circumstances of the case. The functions of such higher co-ordinating structures are known on their subjective side by the name of Intellect. Like all other portions of the sentient system the organs of the Intellect are liable to normal and moderate exercise, subjectively cognized as pleasurable, or to abnormal and excessive exercise, subjectively cognized as painful.

It was necessary in the last chapter to touch slightly upon a few of these phenomena, because the central and peripheral organs of sight are more closely connected with intelligence, genetically and actually, than any others. But we shall have to enter a little more fully here into the pleasures and pains of the Intellect, regarded as a separate element of Æsthetic Feeling. And first, in accordance with our usual plan, we will glance briefly at those emotional phenomena of Intellect which do not attain the æsthetic level.

Acutely painful feelings of intellectual exercise are rare or unknown, as might indeed be expected from the peculiarly secluded position of the organs concerned, which almost precludes the possibility of direct disintegrative action. Intellectual pains are mostly those of fatigue from over use, and of effort or wasteful and ineffectual attempts at complex co-ordinations. The only one among them which ever rises to any great height is that of perplexity; and even this, unless intensified by the affection of fear, is scarcely more than a mere discomfort.

Intellectual pleasures, on the other hand, are common, and often reach considerable distinctness. They arise either from the normal and easy exercise of the structures concerned, in which case the feeling is comparatively faint in pleasurable character, if not absolutely neutral; or from the sudden successful performance of a co-ordination which has for some time baffled the energies concerned, in which case the feeling is often acutely gratifying, and is known as a sense of triumph, pride, power, or exultation. When these latter pleasures are aroused in connexion with the immediate practical ordering of our conduct,—as in the discovery of a path, the settlement of a business difficulty, the invention of a piece of mechanism which has long engaged our faculties,—they are too obviously conducive to useful ends for admission into the æsthetic class. Even when their influence upon practice is only remote,—as in solving a mathematical problem, probing a knotty psychological fallacy, or effecting a physical discovery,—the pleasure is too much alloyed with painful exercise in the pursuit and with ulterior practical aims, to be regarded as æsthetic. It is only the fainter form of pleasure arising from the easy working of the intellectual mechanism which ever becomes a true æsthetic element; and even among these feelings only a comparatively circumscribed number can properly be included in that class. Let us see what is the cause of this special limitation.

If we visit a great city, a zoological garden, a manufactory of glass or hardware, we derive considerable intellectual gratification from the various objects or processes which we observe. Difficulties are solved, unusual combinations are exercised, new facts are noticed, and old ones receive a fresh significance: all of which functional changes are obviously of the pleasurable sort. But the resulting gratification is not necessarily æsthetic. On the other hand, if we visit a beautiful park, an art gallery, a cathedral, the intellectual feelings aroused are immediately recognized as belonging to the æsthetic class. The main difference is this: in the first set of cases the component sensuous factors may be beautiful or ugly indiscriminately, and the intellectual impression is that of useful and interesting knowledge; in the second set of cases, the component sensuous factors are in themselves beautiful, and the intellectual impression is that of immediate and disinterested pleasure. So that there are two necessary principles which must govern every æsthetic intellectual pleasure: first, its sensuous elements must themselves be beautiful; and, second, it must be remote from all ulterior aims. We may be looking at the most lovely prospect in Europe, but if we are scrutinizing it for the purpose of settling the road to our hotel, of determining trigonometrically the height of a mountain, or of reconnoitring an enemy's position in the valley, we derive no æsthetic pleasure from the intellectual processes involved. If, on the contrary, we are surveying it for the purpose of taking in its various beautiful points, and of consciously realizing the emotions it arouses, our intellectual enjoyment is truly æsthetic. In short, intellectual exercise is æsthetic only when it is employed on æsthetic objects for an æsthetic purpose. A few examples will make this clearer.

§ 2. *Æsthetic Feelings connected with the Exercise of the Intellect.*

We have already seen that order and symmetry are elements of many æsthetic totals, and we have allowed that the pleasure derived from them is intellectual in character. Now when order obviously subserves some useful end, or when we are contemplating the end which it subserves, we derive from it a purely practical pleasure. But when it is merely cognized as order-in-the-abstract, without reference to any special end, then the intellectual feeling reaches the necessary disinterestedness of æsthetic pleasure. Thus we may admire the regularity and ingenuity with which the parts of a steam-engine are put together; but as the parts are not in themselves beautiful, and as their purpose is obviously utilitarian, our admiration is not artistic. But when we recognize the symmetry of columns, arches, and windows in a noble building, we recognize it not only as admirable but also as beautiful; because each part is separately an æsthetic sensuous object, and the whole is put together with an æsthetic purpose.*

Next to the intellectual pleasure of symmetry may be placed that of skill in handicraft, which forms so large an element in the gratification derived from the imitative arts. Here, too, the same distinction will be observed. When we are pleased with the perfection of any useful article—a knife, a coat, or a lock—because it will be of ulterior benefit to ourselves or others, the feeling is non-æsthetic; when we notice that much manipulation has been bestowed upon any object in order merely that it may be beautiful, the admiration for the skill displayed becomes an additional æsthetic factor. Thus we may admire smooth and polished surfaces, true-fitting joints, and delicate adjustments, even in machinery. It is delightful to watch the perfect action of a great marine engine, as its cranks turn so powerfully and yet so gracefully at the end of each excursion. But in these cases the pleasure is too obviously connected with a useful end. When, however, the object aims merely at being æsthetically beautiful, as in painting or sculpture, the pleasure felt in fine workmanship is greatly enhanced. Hence, in part, the gratification of polish and glossiness, of variety

* In Mr. Herbert Spencer's Essay on *Use and Beauty* will be found a full account of this relation. I fear I have hardly given enough prominence in parts of my book to the general principle which he there lays down.

and detail, of fine lace and intricate carving. We even transfer the feeling to natural objects, which we figure to ourselves as the result of intelligent design, and compare with mere human standards, so infinitely inferior, admiring the exquisite finish of leaves and flowers, of daintily-fluted shells, and embossed sea-urchins, of many-sided crystals and convoluted coral. And when the microscope reveals to us the wonderful perfection of minute structure in organic bodies or crystalline forms, a new world of intellectual pleasure is laid open before us. We are lost in astonishment, awe, and delight at the myriad facets of an insect's eye, the painted scales of a butterfly's wing, the marvellous symmetry of a tiny flower, and the exquisite architecture of a spangled snow-flake. At each moment we compare their delicacy with the roughness which characterizes even the finest productions of man's hand, the jagged and rugged needle-point, the coarse matting of a cambric handkerchief, the clotted pigment of an oil painting. But though the imperfection of our instruments prevents us from ever rivalling nature in her minute handicraft, we must remember that human skill forms in every case the *point de départ* from which we judge the outer universe.

Here, too, may be noticed our objection to all imitations which fall short of the original in finish and workmanlike skill. Cut glass has a sharp and crystalline edge; when imitated by pressing, the angles are rounded and indefinite, and the lines of junction in the mould are distinctly visible. In machine-made lace or embroidery we miss the delicacy of the hand-made originals. Photographs, where the sun does all the work, are a poor substitute for paintings or steel engravings. Plaster-of-Paris images show at once their hasty and inartistic manufacture. Personal labour bestowed upon any artistic product is never thrown away. Every little touch which betrays the loving care of the artist, is duly noticed and appreciated.

Again, in viewing natural scenery, if the various objects which compose it are tame and monotonous, the absence of intellectual excitement co-operates with the sensuous dullness to produce the feeling of tedium. On the other hand, if the objects are numerous and diversified, besides the variety of sensuous stimulation, we have abundant exercise for the intellect in classifying and recognizing the mutual relations of river, lake, and mountain, castle, church, and abbey, sea and cloud, ship and steamer, deer and swan. To this head we may consequently refer part of the discomfort in monotony, and pleasure in variety, which is further aided by emotional elements of more complex kinds. As a special case, it may be noticed that one main difference between an architectural work and a bit of mason-building is the superior amount of intellectual exercise afforded by the former. Our previous instances of the mid-ocean or the desert, compared with a wide and well-filled landscape, may here again receive mention.

So, too, ornamentation in art or manufactures depends largely for its effect upon the intellectual elements. This is especially noticeable in fictile products. Interest in the design helps out the mere sensuous pleasures of form and colour.

It would be easy to extend this list greatly, and to enumerate many other species of intellectual feelings which may be classed as æsthetic, but I purposely refrain from doing so; partly because sufficient examples will be adduced in later chapters; but partly and more especially because I believe far too great prominence has been hitherto assigned to this order of feelings, under the influence of certain previous writers on Æsthetics, to the manifest neglect of the much more important sensuous elements. I feel convinced that every Æsthetic Feeling, though it may incidentally contain intellectual and complex emotional factors, has necessarily for its ultimate and principal component, pleasures of sense, ideal or actual, either as tastes, smells, touches, sounds, forms, or colours. And I have consequently devoted the larger part of my work to illustrating and enforcing this view; giving only a minor degree of attention to those æsthetic elements which have already been more than sufficiently worked out by others.

It is for a similar reason that I have chosen the title of the present chapter, regarding the office of the Intellect essentially as an *intervention;* that is to say, as supplementary, not as fundamental. It combines sensuously-beautiful factors, so as to yield a synthetic whole more beautiful than all its separate parts. But without the originally æsthetic components, its exercise cannot yield an æsthetic result.

CHAPTER IX.

THE IDEAL.

§ 1. *Mental Pleasures and Pains.*

HITHERTO we have only concerned ourselves with the pleasures and pains of unmistakably bodily origin. Every one of those which we have yet examined is the immediate reflex in consciousness of an existing nervous state. We have seen that the pains of burns and bruises, of bitter tastes and disagreeable smells, of discordant notes and inharmonious colours, or of excessive intellectual labour, are each traceable to an actual present disintegration or waste of nervous tissue. We have observed, similarly, that the pleasure of bodily exercise and field sports, of sweet tastes and agreeable perfumes, of musical combinations and delicate harmonies of shade, or of healthy intellectual activity, are each referable to the due stimulation, at the moment of perception, of structures in a high state of nutrition, ready for the performance of their proper functions. But there is another class of pleasures and pains which we usually call *ideal* or *mental*, and which we are apt to regard as having a less intimate connexion with our nervous organisation.

We have often alluded to them already, without attempting any explanation; and we must now see how far, if at all, we can bring them into accordance with our main principle by showing that the pleasurable feelings of this class correspond to normal performances of function in over-fed and under-worked nervous structures, and that the painful ones are concomitants either of actual disintegration or of excessive and wasteful nervous action.

On searching about for some clue to guide us through this difficult and dangerous labyrinth, we are struck by the fact that a large number of these pleasures and pains, though not apparently connected with due stimulation or destructive action at the actual moment of perception, are yet so connected by anticipation. I allude to the whole class of feelings which involve the phenomenon of pleasurable or painful expectation, roughly expressed as Hopes and Fears. In their elementary form, hope is the expectation of some pleasant sensation; fear, the expectation of some painful one. Now of course the sensations so expected will, when actually present, correspond to a normal stimulation of the nerves in the one case, and a destructive attack upon them in the other. But the new peculiarity introduced into the case, and that which gives it its special interest, is this: that the mere anticipation, as well as the actuality, is in the first instance pleasurable, and in the last disagreeable. Not only does a child derive gratification from the taste of a bun and pain from the smart of a whipping; but it is also pleased by the *promise* of a bun and frightened by the *threat* of a whipping. If we can succeed in explaining these most elementary cases, we shall have found a safe starting-point for our theory of pleasure and pain in the Ideal.

Before attempting the analysis of these states of feeling, however, it may be well to show that they form a portion of that general consensus of the organism on which we have already so often dwelt. It will clearly be for the advantage of the individual that the expectation of pleasure should be pleasurable, for it will then be stimulated to take the proper steps for obtaining the actuality: and equally desirable that the expectation of pain should be painful, for it will then be stimulated to take the proper steps for avoiding the actuality. But this correspondence is of a much more subtle kind than that coarse and immediate one which we noticed in the case of the lower senses. There, by a contrivance closely analogous to reflex action, whatever was to be ultimately destructive to the body was seen to set up premonitory destructive action—cognised as pain—in the first structures with which it was brought into contact, and so to induce cessation of activity or energetic antagonism, as the needs of the case demanded: and, similarly, whatever was to be ultimately beneficial to the body was seen to set up anticipatory normal stimulation—cognised as pleasure—in the first structures with which it was brought into contact, and so to induce continuance of the action till the point of satisfaction was reached. In these higher cases, however, the process is more closely akin to that of volitional activity, because the pleasure or pain is not immediately present to the senses, but is mediately suggested by means of the intellect. Hence they imply a much more complex nervous organization, and much more complicated relations of nervous ganglia, than the correspondence of the lower senses. It is mainly through the organs of sight and hearing that we obtain that information as to the probable future which gives rise to the state of Expectation, either in its emotionally neutral forms, or in its aspects as Hope and Fear. It is mainly through previous experience and the nerve-connexions so functionally established that we interpret the indications yielded us by the senses into premonitions of pleasure and pain. And this process obviously implies the existence and use of those higher co-ordinating structures whose functions are cognised in consciousness as intellect, so that we may expect intellectual phenomena to enter largely into the explanation of our present difficulty.

Among the intellectual processes which may throw a little light upon our question, the most important is that of Attention. It is a well-known fact that out of the various sense-stimulants which continually assail our organs, and which may give rise to impressions known as sights, sounds, smells, tastes, touches, and organic sensations, a vast majority are never consciously cognised at all, while of the remainder a large portion float upon the border-land between consciousness and the unconscious, only a very small number being clearly and distinctly cognised in the foreground of psychical existence. For example, in the visual field, we are generally only conscious at any single moment of a comparatively small central area upon which the eyes are definitely focussed; while the periphery of the field is not present to consciousness at all, and the intermediate portion is half cognised and half unregarded. If we wish to take in the whole field at a glance, as in viewing a beautiful prospect, we are obliged to move the eyes rapidly through their greatest possible sweep, converging them upon all the points separately in very quick succession. Similarly with Hearing. Our ears are constantly receiving aerial impulses from moving bodies in the neighbourhood, such as the ticking of the clock, the sound of the wind, the crackling of the fire, the hum of voices in adjacent rooms, the tread cf footsteps in the street; yet, as a rule, we are utterly unconscious of more than one of these stimuli at a time, or even of them all together. But we can at any moment, by an exercise of the faculty which we call Attention, converge our psychical being upon any one of these sense-stimulants. Thus out of the whole possible number present upon any given occasion, we may specially observe the face of the dial or the ticking of the clock. Of course part of this phenomenon consists in a purely physical alteration in the direction of our organs; as when in the acts of looking and listening we converge and focus the eyes, or tighten the membranes of the ear to the desired degree. But there is another much subtler operation which composes the act of Attention proper. What is this? I think we can hardly fail to answer, if we are consistent physiological psychologists, somewhat after the following fashion. Consciousness, which, as Mr. Herbert Spencer has pointed out, always tends to assume a serial form, is most probably all but exclusively associated in the higher grades of life with the highest co-ordinating centres possessed by each particular grade. It always tends to relegate every minor and automatic function to lower and unconscious organs. Now, though it has never yet attained the complete serial form, it has succeeded in disembarrassing itself of the chief necessary vital functions, such as respiration, digestion, and the circulatory process. Moreover, in the higher mammals, and far more in man, it has to a great extent managed to get rid of the vast majority of sense-impressions. In other words, it seems probable that human consciousness mainly or entirely resides in those higher co-ordinating structures which are the seat of Intellect. To these, the central organs of sensation constantly but by no means universally transmit their disturbances. When the higher co-ordinating structures are occupied in transforming or correlating such transmitted energies, we are in a state of Attention to our sense-impressions; as in the case of observing the dial, or listening to the tick of the clock But when the external stimulus only transmits its disturbance to the central organ of sensation, while the higher co-ordinating centres are engaged upon a different order of functions, we are then said to be in a state of Reflexion, and inattentive to our sense-impressions. Between these two extremes we may have any number of intermediate and alternating states; and, moreover, we may at any moment be attentive to any one portion of the total possible field of stimulation rather than to another; that is to say, the higher co-ordinating structures may be occupied with any one transmitted disturbance rather than another. To take some extreme instances; the higher organs may, under certain circumstances, be so exclusively concerned with their own internal action, and so little interfered with by external disturbances, as to become wholly unconscious of sense-impressions; in which case we are said to be *absorbed in thought*. But even in this state of pre-occupation, any violent and sudden sense-stimulant, such as the roar of a cannon, a flash of lightning, a shooting pain, or an unexpected shaking, communicates its disturbance at once, and forcibly interrupts the regular course of consciousness. Yet men occasionally, under circumstances of great internal activity, are actually unconscious even of the most intense sense-stimulants, as when a soldier in the heat of action is not aware of receiving a wound, or a person in deep grief is unconscious of the most pressing personal danger. The energies which correspond objectively to the main stream of consciousness are so disproportionately greater than the incident energies which correspond to the sense-stimulation, that the latter produce no perceptible change of direction in the total current. So, to sum up, we may conclude that while the automatic vital functions are all but wholly unconnected with consciousness, only adding to its sum in a few morbid conditions;—and while the functions of the sense-organs are intermittently connected with consciousness, sometimes obtruding upon it violently, but generally forming only one of its subordinate elements;—the functions of the higher co-ordinating nervous centres *are* consciousness itself, every other nervous function being only definitely cognised when brought into relation with that system of energies in the higher organs which constitutes the psychical life.*

Let us now apply these views to the two simple cases of Hope and Fear already cited. In children the higher co-ordinating centres have not yet come into full play, and those which work at all are mostly engaged in dealing directly with immediate sense-impressions. If, then, we promise a child a bun, what is the consequence? The notion of the pleasure to come is vividly suggested, and monopolizes the field of consciousness. There is a nascent stimulation of all the nervous structures concerned, and a series of actions are set up, tending more or less towards the realization of the pleasure. If we make the promise an immediate one, and attach any simple condition (such as the giving of a kiss or the utterance of some easy formula, like "ta"), the condition is carried out hastily and with empressement, and a speedy realization is demanded. The higher co-dinating centres have duly accommodated the means to the end. Here we have an easy unimpeded working of the

* It may be objected to the account of Attention here given that it does not attempt to explain what most people mean by that word at all; that is, it deals with natural or primitive Attention, not with the artificial or acquired faculty. To this I would answer that nothing more is required for my purpose. And, indeed, in the majority of phrases Attention bears the meaning here assigned it, though oddly enough the other idea is the one called up by the word in isolation. The phenomenon of strained Attention, though a very interesting one, is confined to the small class of men who have to undertake unpleasant studies for the sake of an ulterior object; and as they are just the class who feel most interest in mental operations, it has come about that this very abnormal case is usually taken as a type of the whole phenomenon; just as in the free-will controversy the unusual but striking example of deliberation has been usually posited as the typical instance of volitional action.

nervous mechanism of intelligence, directed towards an action ultimately desirable for the organism as a whole. And the corresponding feeling in consciousness is, not exactly a pleasure, but what we may call a state of *Enjoyment.* On the other hand, when we threaten a whipping, the notion of pain to come is suggested with equal vividness, and alike monopolizes consciousness. A stimulus is communicated to the higher nervous organs, but its effect is to produce nascent efforts to escape the threatened infliction. If some condition is attached by observing which the penalty may be avoided, it is complied with, and the disagreeable feeling passes away. But if no such outlet offers itself, the result is an exhausting struggle on the part of the higher co-ordinating centres to bring about the desired end; and this cannot be effected, because no appropriate channel is opened. The fruitless effort has for its correlative in consciousness a feeling which is not exactly a pain, but which we may call a state of *Distress.* And if the infliction threatened is one relatively very severe, the waste is long and continuous, and the monopoly of consciousness by the distress reaches a pitch which we name abject terror. So that often "fear is more pain than is the pain it fears." The two classes of feelings, Hopes and Fears, thus described may be taken as simple types of mental pleasures and pains generally, or, as they may better be termed, of Enjoyments and Distresses.

Of course it would have been easy to choose finer and more imposing examples of the feelings here examined, such as the anticipation of pleasure in the return after long absence of a dear friend, or the agony felt at the apprehended loss of a beloved relative. But there are many reasons for preferring the simpler and more elementary case. In the first place, its explanation is shorter and demands less reference to complex emotional phenomena. Again, it only involves such pleasures and pains of simple sensation as we have already accounted for. And, lastly, it is not open to the charge so often and so unjustly brought against the analysis of our higher mental functions, that it is a deliberate attempt to degrade what is noblest in man by referring it to the basest origin. But if, in the above sketch, we substitute the expectation of emotional gratification or emotional distress for the anticipation of sensuous pleasure or sensuous pain, the explanation here attempted will equally well cover such more complex instances. And we must recollect that the actual emotions themselves are pleasurable or the opposite simply because they are normal or abnormal exercises of function in certain structures hereditarily adapted to subserve their special office.

§ 2. *Happiness and Misery.*

We have seen in the last section that the life of man, the most highly developed organism inhabiting this planet, is not wholly made up on its emotional side of the mere pleasures and pains of the moment. As he progresses in intelligence, so is he always widening his emotional horizon, and fore-seeing with ever increasing vividness the pleasures and pains of a more and more distant future. The lamb that sports in the pasture, unconscious of the cruel knife that will so soon cut short his days, is a subject of envy to the poets: but this very unconsciousness is a source of weakness to its species, since that race must in the long run survive which most clearly fore-sees all the dangers and all the possibilities of enjoyment contained in the remotest future. So we find a constant progress of fore-thought with increasing age in the individual and the species. The emotional life of children and savages is chiefly confined to the immediate present. Pleasures and pains promised or threatened for to-morrow seem too far off to force themselves into the thread of consciousness. But with the increase of age and intelligence, the pleasures and pains of the future grow to greater prominence. Small incidents of the moment do not obtrude so violently upon consciousness, which is rather occupied with more general and more complicated co-ordinations. This particular pudding, that particular scratch, become of less importance than the main question how to procure food, clothing, shelter, how to avoid death, hunger, cold, for many days to come. In this way there arise at last the wider conceptions of *Happiness* and *Misery*, in contrast to the simpler ones of pleasure and pain. A happy life is one not merely made up of momentary pleasures, sensuous and emotional, but free from serious anxiety about the future, and filled with anticipations of enjoyment. A miserable life is its exact opposite. Accordingly, happiness, not mere pleasure, is the end at which civilized men aim for themselves and those they love. In beings endowed with highly-developed nervous systems, consciousness is chiefly occupied with remote possibilities of pleasure and pain. To see one's path smooth before one, to have a home, food, a fixed income, a wife, a family, and a sufficiency of health and worldly goods to make them and one's self comfortable for life, gives a background of contentment on which the individual pleasures of the moment can firmly base themselves. A few headaches or an occasional slight cross in business do not seriously interfere with the course of such a life. On the other hand, to be invalided, to have no home, or the prospect of losing one, to be in want of a fixed income, and to have one's personal fears increased by the awful anticipation of suffering for those whom one loves, gives a background of wretchedness which no immediate sense-allurements can overcome. Consciousness is too deeply engaged with the difficulties of co-ordinating the impracticable to allow the intrusion of such minor pleasures upon its sombre woof.

It is obvious that in the first of these cases the highest nervous functions are carried on with the greatest ease and simplicity, while in the second a certain struggle exists in which the higher nervous tissues are wastefully consumed. This fact has been actually proved by the observation that after periods of severe mental perplexity the products of nerve-waste in the excretions appear in largely increased quantities. Hence we see why mental pleasure is felt to be akin to bodily pleasure, and mental pain to bodily pain. At the same time we see the reason of the distinction between them: the bodily pains being sharper and more clearly marked; the mental, rather distinguished by that characteristic which the Greeks well called ἀπορία, a sense of utter inability to escape from a difficult and untenable position. And conversely with the bodily and mental pleasures: the former are characterized by acute and momentary stimulation; the latter, by a constant and placid undercurrent of consciousness, flowing easily along unimpeded channels.

§ 3. *Ideal Æsthetic Feelings.*

The reader may perhaps have enquired to what purpose this long introduction has tended. That question we may now hope to answer. It is clear that we cannot be concerned in the present work with those mental pleasures and pains which are anticipatory of bodily states in close connexion with vital functions, such as the hopes of food and shelter, or the fears of cold, hunger, and enemies. But if there is any class of emotional states, purely ideal, and not connected with necessary vital functions, then they will answer to our definition of Æsthetic Feelings, and may form the elements of a fine art. Such a class is actually found in the mental pleasures and pains which are exclusively employed in Poetry and Romance, and which also form large components of Painting and Sculpture. Let us consider what is their origin and explanation.

We have seen above the nature of ordinary Hopes and Fears. But besides the class which consist of immediate anticipations of pleasure or pain, and the class which give the undercurrent of brightness or gloom to consciousness at large, there is a third class less directly anticipatory, and recognized as involving a much greater element of uncertainty, which we call *day-dreaming* or *building castles in the air* on the one hand, and *taking trouble at interest* on the other. The last phenomenon is a special and we may almost say a morbid one: it does not aid us in averting the actuality; and so, in healthy organisms it is banished from consciousness as soon as it appears. But the other and pleasanter form is a cheap and easy amusement, giving free play to certain of the faculties without much risk of serious ultimate disappointment. Its rise will clearly throw some light upon the ideal pleasures generally.

First, we must notice that no sharp line can be drawn between the ordinary faculty of fore-thought, by which we co-ordinate our plans for the future, and the more fanciful faculty which we employ in day-dreaming. Whenever we are about to take an important step in life we not only think over its immediate results, and arrange for the proximate future, but we also reflect upon all the possibilities of happiness which it involves, and allow the attention to dwell upon them rather than upon their opposites. Before marriage, we talk over the arrangements of our house, our probable trips and excursions, our domestic enjoyments, our visits from friends and relations, with all the other delights which open temptingly before our exuberant fancies. On entering a University, taking up a profession, moving to a new sphere of life, attaining a dignity, we similarly form our plans for the future, not only so far as we can actually calculate, but into the remoter regions of mere conjecture. Such building of castles in the air, however, though pleasurable enough, does not rise to the æsthetic level, and for this reason, that it is too monopolist, too closely connected with our own future happiness. We are ourselves the centres of every such dream, and its main pleasure consists in the notion of its possible realization in our own persons.

Sometimes, though our individual selves still form the nucleus round which the story gathers, we cut the link which connects our dream with reality, and imagine ourselves placed in all but impossible positions. At one time we come unexpectedly into large fortunes; at another we are made Prime Ministers or Commanders-in-Chief; and we then work out our course of action in these exalted positions. Occasionally we depart still further from possibility, so as not only to idealize the future but to make the past course of our lives different from actual fact. But in all these cases we still, by an illusion of fancy, preserve our personal identity, and think of the rich and handsome hero in these flights of imagination as a phase of our known selves. It is to be noticed that these unreal dreams are distinguished from the former class by the fact that their realization is not expected, and is often actually self-contradictory. Hence they are indulged in chiefly when we have no opportunity for the extended exercise of our faculty of planning for the future. At those periods of our life when the higher co-ordinating portions of the brain are occupied in arranging definite designs which are to be carried into practical execution, as at all special crises of our personal history, we do not feel the need for these wider excursions. If we draw upon the fancy at all, we connect our day-dreams with our actual plans, and to some extent provide for the fulfilment of both together. But in moments of occasional recoil from the monotonous course of humdrum business life, we give free play to the otherwise unexercised faculty in speculations which have no bearing upon our immediate actions. Especially in childhood and youth, when our co-ordinating powers are inadequate to grapple with the difficulties of real life, and when our parents take upon themselves the serious business of directing our future, we employ the nascent faculty on wild schemes of future success, military, practical, or amatory. And, in later life, when unhappy circumstances lead to the constant monopolizing of consciousness by unpleasant actualities or fears and doubts for the immediate future, we sometimes escape for a time from the wretchedness so caused and obtain a momentary relief by conjuring up delusive pictures of imaginary happiness.

It is not only in these larger and more conspicuous instances that pleasure can be derived from the idea in the absence of the actuality. Even the special sense-pleasures can to some extent be represented ideally with a gratifying effect. We may notice that people, compelled by some unusual circumstances to live on hard fare, as in a siege, a shipwreck, or an African expedition, often derive pleasure from talking over the dishes they will indulge in upon their return to civilization and plenty. So the poor and those suffering from severe illness picture to themselves the various sense-pleasures they might derive from money or health. And, without multiplying instances, we may say generally, that whatever gives us pleasure in the actuality carries with it a faint tinge of pleasure in the idea.

The reason for this is not wholly confined, I believe, to the action of the central organs. It seems probable that every idea, besides involving a stimulation of the nervous centre or group of centres in which the corresponding actuality is cognised, also implies a certain amount of communicated disturbance in the fibres attached. Directing the attention to any part of the body has a noticeable effect upon its vaso-motor nerves: the sensation of itching and the blush are conspicuous examples. Sexual images rouse physical excitement in the correlated organs. The sight of agreeable food, especially when hungry, makes the mouth water. Suggestions of nauseating ideas bring on sickness in weak states of the stomach. Indeed, we may regard the idea in every case as an incomplete form of the actuality. Hence we may conclude with great probability that when any body of nerve-fibres and their central terminal organs have been long deprived of their natural stimulant, and are consequently in a high state of nutrition, they will derive a certain amount of pleasure from that centrally-initiated stimulation which is cognised in consciousness as ideal, though not so large an amount as they would derive from that more normal peripherally-initiated stimulation which is cognised in consciousness as actual sensation. And we find as a matter of experience that any ideal pleasure is greatest when we have been longest deprived of the actuality.

Here, then, we reach at last the explanation of Ideal Æsthetic Pleasure which we have so long been seeking. When the gratification derived from the exercise of nervous organs in the ideal form is connected in thought with our own personality and made part of an imaginary programme of our future lives, the pleasure is too monopolist to reach the æsthetic level. But when that gratification is the product of exercise unconnected in thought with our own personality, and wholly cut off from actuality, it becomes a subject for æsthetic employment, both in poetical and pictorial representation.

With this psychological origin for the sister arts of Poetry and Painting is inextricably mixed up another and more purely intellectual one,—that of plot-interest. The youngest child is pleased with a story, and finds an outlet for its budding intelligence in following the incidents of a nursery rhyme or a fairy tale. If one offers to draw for it upon a slate, it immediately proposes a subject for dramatic treatment;—a man shooting a bird, or a lady riding on horseback. From this common starting-point of the child and the savage diverge the various forms of Poetry and Romance, of historical and genre Painting. The earliest literature consists of tales and ballads; the earliest pictorial art represents the king in battle, the offering to the gods, or those domestic operations with which we are so familiar in Egyptian remains. From the union of these two pleasures, the intellectual and the ideal, flow the various forms of higher æsthetic enjoyment. The part which each bears in the complex total varies, of course, with the particular style of art. Plot-interest is of greatest importance in Romance, narrative Poetry, and historical Painting; ideal sensuous or emotional feeling predominates in descriptive or lyrical Poetry, landscape Painting, and Music.

A few of the simpler instances chosen from general literature will make this clear. The fairy-tales in which children delight combine a certain element of plot-interest with a much larger proportion of ideal sensuous gratification. The persons with whom the story deals are every one of them kings and queens, princes and princesses. They are all young, beautiful, rich, strong, and happy. Feasting, dancing, and love-making fill up the whole of their existence. There are no lessons, no rainy days, and no whippings in fairy-land; everything is as bright and glorious as it can be. The magical power of the fairies smooths every difficulty and gets rid of every annoyance. Pumpkins turn into gilt carriages and mice into prancing steeds at a single wave of the silver wand. Life moves on through a circle of delights; no serious cares disturb the harmony of existence; and if some great misfortune threatens for a moment, it is at once dispelled by the timely assistance of the supernatural godmother. In the end, the hero and heroine invariably marry and live happily ever afterwards.* The "Arabian Nights" give us an instance in which plot-interest is slightly more conspicuous: but here too there is a profusion of ideal sense-pleasures. Cool sherbets, delicious fruits, gardens perfumed with roses, vocal with nightingales, and peopled by peacocks coloured like the rainbow; palaces filled with gold, silver, and precious stones; sultanas of surpassing beauty; harems crowded with the fairest Circassians; troops of obsequious servants, and caravans laden

* If it be objected that the historical growth of fairy-tales from degraded myths does not bear out this view, I answer that though such is undeniably their origin, they have been gradually adopted, in the course of ages, to their altered purpose of yielding simple imaginative pleasure to undeveloped minds.

with spices, dates, and perfumes;—these are the staple of the entertainment, interspersed with marvellous adventures and hair-breadth escapes. The poetry and romance of Chivalry contain similar elements,—jousts and tournaments, richly caparisoned steeds and ladies gaily dight, feasts and minstrelsy in hall or bower, with all the paraphernalia of courtly pageant and knightly adventure, arranged to suit the tastes of mediæval readers, and with plot-interest still further developed and sustained. Lastly, in most cultivated literatures a considerable differentiation takes place, and we get as distinct forms Romance, which depends almost entirely upon its connected story, and Poetry, which consists of the purely æsthetic elements sifted and combined into a harmonious whole.

But it is only the lowest forms of art which rely mainly or exclusively upon sensuous gratifications even in their idealised form. The fairy-tales of our childhood and the chivalric romances of our youth pall upon our adult imagination. We still require the same sensuous elements in our pictures and our poems, but we require that they should be subordinated to another order of pleasures which we recognise as higher and more ennobling. These are the ideal emotions which deserve for their exposition a short separate section.

§ 4. *Ideal Complex Emotional Feelings.*

To trace the origin of the manifold complex Emotions in the human organism would be a task clearly beyond the sphere of the present work. However interesting and tempting such an enquiry may appear, we must be content here to take for granted the existence in man of a large number of developed complex Emotions, such as the maternal, domestic, and social affections, the love of country and the sentiment of religious veneration, whose normal exercise upon their proper objects yields the ordinary gratification of function in fully-nurtured structures. All that we shall have to do here is to show that besides the immediate and actual pleasures of real exercise, these faculties are capable of yielding ideal pleasures from their application to imaginary objects.

Fortunately this is a comparatively easy matter. The structures upon which these feelings depend being always stimulated, not immediately by combinations of external energies, but mediately through the action of the higher coordinating centres upon the disturbances transmitted by such incident energies, it naturally follows that they may be excited almost as easily by the ideal suggestion of their proper object as by its actual presence. And such we find by positive experience to be the case.

In youth the amatory passion (amongst civilized men) constantly manifests itself at first in the form of ideal cravings. With women who happen never to have attached the emotion to a particular person, it often expends itself upon ideal heroes, upon pets, or even upon plants and flowers. Sometimes, too, it takes a more abnormal outlet in a general tendency towards the romantic, or in a strengthening of the devotional feelings. Hence the indulgence of sentimental friendships among girls, or the impulse towards conventual life. Similarly with the maternal instinct. Unmarried girls, especially of mature age, manifest a deep interest in the babies of other women, and are never so happy as in tending and nursing them. Even little children delight in the playful exercise of maternal solicitude towards dolls and kittens. Both these feelings are carried into the purely ideal sphere by painting and poetry. The domestic and social affections in like manner can be ideally gratified by allusion or pictorial representation. The malevolent feelings display themselves in kindred shapes. Burning in effigy an unpopular person; shaking the fist and grinding the teeth behind an enemy's back; lampooning, caricaturing, or abusing an adversary, are common examples. Defacing a statue or picture, and hacking at an imaginary figure, carry the realization a point further. Satirical poetry and political cartoons are the artistic outcome of these impulses. The emotion of combat, so deeply rooted in our race, is gratified by ideal representations. Boys' sports, like prisoner's-base, foot-ball, and rounders, all contain a pugnacious element. Mr. Herbert Spencer has pointed out that antagonism is an essential part of most games, appearing even in chess, whist, or billiards. Patriotism is at once stimulated and gratified by historical or rhetorical descriptions of our country's greatness, and by poems like the Charge of the Light Brigade, or paintings of Waterloo and Trafalgar. When we talk of Marathon and Thermopylæ, we are all Greek for the moment, transferring our allegiance to the wider interests of culture, freedom, and civilization. And as we advance in breadth of moral sympathies, we find the higher arts striving faintly and tentatively after the embodiment of those sentiments which are most in harmony with the highest aims and aspirations of the race. The older appeals to the monopolist senses, to the selfish feelings, to the narrower sympathies of class, and race, and nationality, and creed, are yielding place, we may hope, at least in our poetry and possibly even in our imitative arts, to the nobler sentiments of all-embracing humanitarianism. It is in this way and in this way only that art can fully deserve those eulogistic titles which it so often receives. So long as it remains merely a means for the gratification of the senses, without strengthening the higher consonant aims of life, it can only claim to rank as the most exquisite and self-sustaining among the selfish enjoyments. When it rises to be the handmaid of ethical purpose, it may worthily take its place beside the grandest products of human development, Science and Right, having as its object to enrich and beautify our lives by tuning us unconsciously into harmony with whatever is noblest in nature or in man.

CHAPTER X.

THE IMITATIVE ARTS.

§ 1. *The Origin of Imitation.*

We have now completed our survey of the separate elements which compose Æsthetic Feelings. But it will help greatly to illustrate our general principles if we take a few of the great synthetic totals, known as works of art, and analytically resolve them into these ultimate factors. Indeed, such an analysis of the highest artistic product, Poetry, is the final goal which we have placed before ourselves in the present treatise. As an introduction to this we may glance first at the Imitative Arts of Painting and Sculpture.

Among the earliest products of human industry revealed to the present generation by archæological research have been found sundry rude imitations of the forms of men or animals, roughly scratched with splinters of flint upon the tusks of the mammoth. In our own day the most civilized races hold annual exhibitions for the display of paintings and statuary, representing scenes of human life or of inanimate nature, skilfully pourtrayed in the richest pigments or exquisitely carved in the finest marble. The question which we have to attack in the present chapter is this: What is the origin of that pleasure which the most savage and the most cultured men alike have always felt in delineating external objects or in observing such delineations by the hands of others? To answer it we must dive a little deeper than hitherto into the volitional sources of artistic production.

We have seen already that the due exercise of the limbs and muscles yields us the ordinary gratification of normal function. But man cannot be satisfied, like the lower animals, with the simple enjoyment of such coarse bodily actions as walking, running, and leaping. He possesses by hereditary transmission a set of highly-developed nervous centres which are adapted for accurately correlating the most varied and delicate muscular actions. The faculties of which these centres are the governing organs constantly require a proper outlet. Hence our inability ever to indulge in that complete state of indolence which is habitual with the lower animals in the intervals of life-serving functions, and which is familiar to us all in the cat and the dog. We are perpetually impelled by our fully-fed nervous centres to be employed upon some kind of occupation. Even in our congeners the monkeys this restless activity is sufficiently noticeable; in the savage it is more intelligently directed to useful ends; and in the civilized man it seeks to vent itself upon some higher object. But when any unusual circumstances, such as a railway-journey, a sea-voyage, or the forced inaction of a waiting-room, prevent us from following our ordinary avocations and deprive us of our common resources in reading and society, we are generally driven to amuse ourselves by some comparatively purposeless exercise of the more delicate organs of correlation. How we do it varies with our temperament. We may whittle a piece of stick into a doll or a tooth-pick; we may cut out figures with a paper and scissors; we may draw pencil sketches on our finger nails; we may fish over the ship's side for sargasso-weed; we may plait the loose ends of the leather window-strap; we may deface the letters on the company's notices; we may carve our initials on the wood-work; we may smoke, bite our nails, or hum a tune; but something or other we *must* do. Under ordinary circumstances adult men have enough to occupy them without such shifts; but women of the upper classes are obliged to expend their superfluous energies on embroidery, wool-work, vitromanie, wood-carving, leather-moulding, and a thousand other quasi-artistic expedients. In short the nervous structures are there, and an appropriate object must be found for them.

Of course all these facts already postulate the series of prior developments by which such complicated organs of correlation have been brought into existence. The function is imperative because the structures exist; and the structures exist because previous function has slowly perfected them. So that these characteristics of civilized man cannot account for the first artistic attempts of the savage. But in the savage too, though to a less extent, there is a necessity for exercising the hands upon comparatively useless work. Just as the eye, whose main functions are at first those of searching for food or mates and anticipating the approach of enemies, must yet expend its energies in viewing countless other objects during its intervals of leisure; so the hands, when not engaged in hunting or fishing, in wattling the hut, polishing the stone hatchet, or framing the bow, will occasionally employ themselves at stray moments in playing with tools and materials. From such leisure employment will arise, mainly by hazard, the earliest forms of that sportive industry which we call art. The artistic feelings, as Schiller hinted and Mr. Herbert Spencer has proved at length, take their origin in the play-instinct.

Give a child a slate and pencil, and allow it to sit down quietly by itself without any suggestion as to what it shall do with them. At first it will be satisfied with making lines and splashes; but after a while it will begin to form a series of marks upon the slate which half by accident bear a remote resemblance to some familiar shape, such as a plate, a rectangular house, or a human profile. The intellect at once seizes upon the resemblance, and there is a pleasurable thrill of recognition, together with an emotional elation of power. The child is incited to a fresh attempt, and this time succeeds a little better. A few trials result in the completion of a formal or conventional representation of the object imitated, which satisfies for a considerable period the imperfect intelligence of the child. For example, a house is symbolized by four moderately straight lines, enclosing a smaller rough rectangle for the door, and two lesser ones for the windows; a profile is represented by a straight forehead, an angular nose, and a re-entrant angle for the mouth, with a circular or oval eye put somewhere above the nose. These symbolical forms are repeated once or twice till they become ingrained in the nervous and muscular systems; and improvements are only very slowly introduced, each one tending itself to be similarly stereotyped in the motor apparatus; just as, in learning to write, we incorporate each new acquisition in our formal style, and so produce what we call *our hand.* Savage and semi-civilized art long continues in this conventional stage; indeed, the symbolical representation is much more easily recognised by savages than the most artistic picture. But while our child is thus gratifying his motor system by the exercise of scrawling, he is also gratifying his perceptive and intellectual system by the constant recognition of similarity. The pleasure of art-production and the pleasure of art-perception grow up side by side.

As with the infant, so with the early development of the race. The first rough design sketched half-unconsciously by the savage with flint or deer-horn will be but a very imperfect representation of the object which it is intended to pourtray. But successive attempts will better the imitation, and will be productive of renewed pride and pleasure in the artist. His fellows will be struck by the skill exhibited, and will derive an intellectual gratification from observing it. For we have seen that the exhibition of skill always pleases us, first in ourselves, and afterwards, sympathetically, in others. This feeling will already have been roused in the manufacture of celts, fish-hooks, and arrow-heads; it will soon extend itself to the new faculty of imitation, and the fortunate artist will be able to give a new pleasure to his admiring follow-tribesmen. Shortly, more truly æsthetic elements will be introduced in bright colouring and graceful forms. Art will gradually select for imitation only what is most beautiful in nature, rejecting all that is ugly, discordant, and base. But many ages will be required for this passage from mere imitation to developed fine art; and it will best be considered in a separate section.

We may note in passing that it is very difficult to draw any sharp line between the two main classes of art, the imitative and the decorative. Originally there is a considerable distinction between the circles and splashes which adorned the rude pottery of primitive man, and the figures which he etched to represent human or animal forms. Indeed, it has been noticed that some tribes of savages exclusively adopt the one system, and some the other. But in the process of time the two become inextricably blended by the introduction of conventional imitative figures into geometrical ornamentation. Most symmetrical patterns at the present day consist of intermediate forms, such as festoons, scrolls, sprays of formal foliage, or grotesque heads of birds and animals. But in the succeeding sections of this chapter we shall only deal with the regular imitative arts in their purest form. They include within themselves all minor developments.

§ 2. *Painting.**

There are four separate kinds of pleasure which Painting may seek to arouse; first, the actual sensuous pleasure of

* The two sections which follow on Painting and Sculpture, I put forward with considerable diffidence. I am a psychologist, not an art-critic, and I am loth to go *ultra crepidam*. Hence I have refrained from quoting special instances, lest my taste should be called in question by those competent to

form and colour; second, the ideal sensuous pleasure of suggested softness, smoothness, musical sound, coolness, warmth, sweetness, or comfort generally; third, the ideal emotional pleasure of the various special sentiments; fourth, the intellectual pleasure of skilful imitation. To all these is sometimes added the other form of intellectual pleasure known as plot-interest. Each of these we must examine seriatim.

The Actual Sensuous Pleasure of form and colour has already been explained, and is of course specially expected in pictorial art. As to *form*, we demand that a painter should choose for his theme beautifully-shaped objects, such as human figures, male or female, in graceful attitudes, nude and exquisitely formed, with rounded limbs, or clothed in flowing drapery, Greek or Roman, Oriental or Florentine; animals like the fawn, the panther, the Arab charger, the swan, and the butterfly; mountain peaks, bossy hills, winding bays; the cataract leaping in an arch from the crag; Naples and Vesuvius, Tivoli and Niagara, the curved horizon of ocean, the thousand inlets of a highland loch; graceful pottery, elegantly-moulded goblets, flagons, and vases, slender beakers and shapely chalices; the domes and minarets of Stamboul, the sweeping arches of Tintern and Poitiers, the columns of Pæstum, the rounded tiers and galleries of the amphitheatre. On the other hand, the painter generally avoids (except for some special effect of colour or contrast)

do so. All I can do is to account to the best of my ability for those feelings which works of art arouse in me personally, and which observation or enquiry have revealed to me as existing in other people. I can deal with them merely as so many known facts, without much reference to the place which they would fill in a graduated scale of æsthetic feelings.

lean, harsh, and angular limbs or features, constrained and graceless clothing, awkward postures and actions; heavy, ungainly, or shapeless animal forms, such as the bear, the cart-horse, the goose, and the slug; flat and monotonous plains; the still ocean unbroken by a winding shore or bluff headland, unrelieved by a ship with bellied sails or a tempest curling the breakers on the beach; straight streets, plain rectangular houses, square windows, and flat façades destitute of arch or column, dome or portico. As to *colour*, we demand sufficient stimulation blended with due relief; warm reds and oranges, not too strong, too massive, or too prominent; delicate toning and harmony; together with variety and fitness for the objects delineated. The drapery of historical paintings is selected with an eye to mixed effectiveness and harmony of hues; sacred subjects, oriental pieces, and scenes of the XVIth, XVIIth, and XVIIIth centuries admit of gayer colouring as well as more graceful shapes than the ordinary incidents of modern life; and amongst the latter, such are generally chosen as will give an opportunity for the introduction of bright female costumes, or else of court and military uniforms, while the present sombre and inartistic dress of men in every-day life almost defies pictorial representation. Landscape of course presents us with all the hues of natural scenery which it would be tedious again to particularize. The choice of "bits" is one of the greatest tests of an artist's natural taste. Autumn and sunset are the chosen seasons of the painter as well as the poet. Reds are far more common in art than in nature, and bright colours are lavished in considerable profusion. In short, all those tints and shapes which please us elsewhere are selected and combined in Painting.

The Ideal Sensuous Pleasure of suggested feelings is plentifully found in Painting. Ease of movement is given in the attitudes of dances, especially such as the minuet and the coranto. Flesh is so represented as to convey the notion of softness and warmth. Satin and velvet, grass and moss, tempt us to stroke them. Glossiness reveals the smooth surface of jet or amber. The glow of a fireside is rendered in such a manner that we almost feel its comfortable warmth. Domestic pieces generally rouse the sense of comfort and happiness. Coolness is suggested by river-side nooks and green fern-clad grottos. Fruit-pieces display grapes and melons, pomegranates and filberts, temptingly before our eyes, till we long to taste their luscious flavour. We can almost smell the roses and the heliotrope; while, as to musical sound, I have seen at least one painting of a throstle in a hawthorn bush, pouring forth its soul in open-mouthed delight, so that the very notes of its song trembled in one's ear.

The Ideal Emotional Pleasure of the various complex sentiments is, however, a much larger component of artistic gratification. It will not be necessary to enter fully into illustrations here, as these sentiments will be treated in extenso under the head of Poetry: but a very few pictorial examples may be briefly run through, for the sake of formal completeness. The emotion of sublimity is given in mountains, crags, the stormy ocean, and the thunder-cloud riven by the bolt: it is also aroused by supernatural beings, of vast and shadowy proportions or Miltonesque vagueness; by palaces and castles, knights and princesses, heroes of gigantic limbs, and all that is antiquated, venerable, or mystic. The painter, once more like the poet, lives mainly in the storied or imagined past.* The religious sentiment is appealed to, in earlier times by pictures of the gods and their doings; under Christian influences, by saints and martyrs, angels and cherubim, tiara'd popes and mitred bishops, the attitude of prayer or praise, the dim cathedral and the village church. The emotion of pity gives us the blind beggar and the wounded soldier, the widowed bride and the fatherless bairn. Here, as elsewhere, love of course forms a main theme, but specification is both difficult and unnecessary. The domestic sentiments are also fully represented by fireside pieces and village scenes. Patriotism and the allied ego-altruistic feelings of military life flood the walls of exhibitions yearly with battle-pieces and loyal demonstrations. Even the purely personal and monopolist pleasures of pride and power may sometimes be imported with effect into artistic works.†

The three classes of pictorial gratification which we have hitherto examined are concerned chiefly with design; the next class, Intellectual Pleasure of Skilful Imitation, is dependent on execution alone. This is the proper pleasure of imitative art. In its coarsest form,—that felt by the child, the savage, and the rustic,—it consists merely in the apprehension of likeness between the representation and the object

* See this point fully worked out in Mr. Herbert Spencer's Essay on *Use and Beauty*.

† The difficult question of the employment in art of *painful* emotions will be considered under the head of Poetry.

represented. In a slightly higher stage, that of the appreciative but uncritical public, it consists in gratification at the workmanship as a whole, apart from any consciousness of the minute skill displayed. In its highest form, as seen in the artist and the trained art-critic, it consists in a rational recognition of the end attained and the means employed for its attainment. In this last case, all the difficulties of a particular scene are accurately comprehended, and the tact and knowledge with which they have been overcome is distinctly observed. The gloss on the satin; the glow of the fire; the bloom on the peach; the transparency of the muslin beneath which the soft shoulder is half hidden, half perceived; the motion of the waterfall; the spray from the angry waves; the trembling of the hand that tries to hide the furtive love-letter:—all these demand the utmost skill, and receive the highest praise when dexterously imitated. Here, too, we must include all the technique of art: the proper use of pigments and vehicles; the knowledge of anatomy, of perspective, of chiaroscuro; the power of grouping and composition; the employment of all that slowly-accumulated science which raises modern art above the rude bas-reliefs of Egypt and Assyria. And just as the marksman alone can fully appreciate a contest at long ranges; just as the billiard-player alone can fully appreciate the skill which makes a break of three hundred, or scores a ten-stroke from a seemingly hopeless leave, by marvellous calculations of side and angle,—so the artist alone can fully appreciate the wonderful art by which a straw stands out in the foreground, a cranny in the wall is filled with moss or stone-crop, and a distant hill is made to loom weirdly through depths of intervening mist. Art thus projects itself even into the appreciation of nature, and every scene is viewed and enjoyed by the painter with a tacit reference to its capabilities for pictorial representation.

Lastly, we may have, in addition to all these varied gratifications, the Intellectual Pleasure of Plot-Interest. A painting may represent a living action and tell its own story. A Greek interior, a Roman domestic group, an incident of the palæstra or the arena, a Venetian love-tale, a page from the stately annals of Florence or Genoa, a scene from Shakespeare or Molière, Goldsmith or Cervantes, a Spanish bull-fight, a village feast in Flanders, a touching sketch of English farmhouse life. In telling the story there is again much scope for artistic skill in face and figure, in delicate shades of emotion and suggestions of inner thought. Some exquisite little touch in the corner of a mouth, or the drooping of an eyelid, is often the making of a picture's fame. Indeed, plot-interest is the element of pleasure which is most strongly felt by the inartistic public. At exhibitions, the crowd collects around the canvas which most vividly tells the most interesting history. Landscapes of marvellous detail and single heads of ideal beauty are mostly left to the admiring eyes of the cognoscenti.

It will thus be seen that Painting, in one or other of its forms, yields us in the highest possible degree that harmonious combination—the maximum of stimulation with the minimum of fatigue—which we saw to be the essence of æsthetic pleasure, and yields it to us in every department of our nature, sensuous, ideal, emotional, and intellectual. All classes of paintings, however, do not equally depend upon all these forms of pleasure. The only one which is necessarily present in every case is the actual sensuous gratification of form and colour, simple and combined, and that of skilful imitation. Landscape depends chiefly upon these. It may also call up ideal sensuous pleasures of coolness, softness, or sweet odour; as in the case of a mossy bank or a new-mown hay-field. Historical paintings add the special emotions of pity, sublimity, or patriotism. They owe much, too, to plot-interest. Genre tells us an amusing or interesting tale, and further appeals to the domestic emotions or the amatory passion. Sacred art is a special study by itself. Military pieces depend for part of their effect upon the combative instincts: they are most popular amongst the most warlike nations. Minor details can be easily filled in by the memory and imagination of the reader.

A few cursory remarks may be added upon the development of pictorial art, viewed from our present psychological standpoint. The earliest attempts of the savage are devoid of any care for harmony of colour or gracefulness of form. Beyond bright and striking hues, the mere pleasure of successful imitation is all that he prizes, and even in that he is satisfied with a very low and conventional standard. A step higher up, Egyptian art delights in the powerful and unusual stimulation of the analytic colours, but does not attempt harmony, shading, or tone. It gives us tolerably accurate representations of men, animals, and plants, *in the abstract*, without reference to special circumstances, emotional expression, perspective, or chiaroscuro. In its arrangement it is strictly symmetrical and conventional. In purpose it is rather religious and governmental than æsthetic, and so it does not appeal to any other sentiments than those which suit its special object. Offerings to the gods, the judgment of the dead, the king capturing a city, the king surveying his prisoners—these are stock specimens of its choice of subjects. Faces and figures exhibit no kind of emotion. A soldier kills or is killed, a king hunts or performs religious ceremonies, with exactly the same wooden attitude, the same stonily indifferent cast of features. Still, to the undeveloped intellects which observed them, these pictures doubtless afforded the gratification of bright colour, comparative skill in imitation, and a certain amount of plot-interest. Assyrian bas-reliefs show, perhaps, a trifle more appreciation for beauty of form, especially in animals. A step above this we may interpolate Chinese art, whose line of development was unconnected with the West. This gives us much improvement in colouring and shading, considerable expression of emotion and life-like attitude, with greater variety of plot-interest; but the emotions aroused are usually low and sometimes (to our ethical feelings) disgusting. The Japanese arrange brilliant colours in very effective combinations; their imitation of trees and animals is good; their landscape is often pretty: and the emotions are represented with much spirit and vigour. To return to the regular line of Western development, classical painting shows us an enormous advance over all that preceded it with that marvellous rapidity which characterizes the whole growth of Hellenic culture. In it we get a sudden yet traceable transition from simple imitative painting to æsthetic art. We see harmonious arrangement of delicately-shaded colours, instead of mere powerful primary stimulation. Exquisite gracefulness in the shape of limbs and arrangement of drapery replaces the straight, stiff contours, the coarse, angular forms of Egyptian painting. The imitation approaches much more nearly to actual life. Figures are naturally grouped in unsymmetrical composition. There is considerable display of plot-interest in the scenes depicted from the beautiful living mythology;—Theseus, the Minotaur, Ariadne, Dionysus and his train; Odysseus, Calypso, the Cyclops, Scylla and her dogs. But even here, all is not perfect. Emotion is very slightly exhibited in the faces; most of them have a calm, statuesque repose. Single figures are managed with great skill; but deeper perspective still baffles the artist, and composition is yet in its infancy. Although the human figure has been emancipated from the trammels of conventionalism, animal shapes, vegetation, and landscape generally, are still formal and unreal. Nevertheless, in Painting, as in every other higher department of human handicraft or intelligence, it was the Hellenes who took the first great step from the material to the spiritual. Egypt had bright colour and amusing imitation; Hellas first introduced that higher æsthetic pleasure which we term distinctively *beauty*. We must pass over Roman painting, which was really Greek in all but the name, and omit the gradual decline of Byzantine art—with its recurrence to primary colours, excessive gilding, and conventional arrangement—as well as the deluge of Western barbarism, and the mediæval love for minute skill in delineation, coupled with want of truthfulness to nature in her wider manifestations. With the earlier Italian revival of art, conventionalism is once more discarded, and the higher pleasures of faithful natural imitation re-instated in the first rank of artistic feeling. Lastly, modern post-Raphaelite painting, departing from the narrow choice of Madonnas, Holy Families, and St. Sebastians, and appealing to the widest possible range of emotions, gives us, in one or other of its special and highly-differentiated forms, every one of the above-enumerated classes of Æsthetic pleasure.*

§ 3. *Sculpture.*†

Some early forms of Sculpture undoubtedly preceded the first attempts at Painting. To carve a grotesque head upon the club or the stick, as savages constantly do, is almost naturally suggested by its shape. The lineal descendants of these rude imitative efforts are still to be seen on our walking sticks, our umbrella handles, and our briar-root pipes. The South Sea Islanders make hideous gods of feathers, and the Africans give a monstrous human shape to clay or soft stone. But that form of art which in its

* For the purposes of this section it has been both impossible and unnecessary to distinguish in the earlier periods between Painting and bas-relief.

† Sculpture I approach with even more diffidence than Painting, partly because of the greater delicacy of the feelings involved, and partly because I am obliged to express opinions which come nearer to the critical level. I do so, however, in all due deference to those whose higher tastes may lead them to differ from my conclusions.

full development we know as Sculpture is not the direct offshoot of these crude artistic beginnings. It is rather a differentiated species of the original mode of painting, practised by the founders of our Western civilization, which, beginning with a single scratched outline, developed at last into coloured bas-relief, having the contour lines incised, and the pigment spread upon the raised portions. From this common beginning, Sculpture gradually progressed through the differentiating stages of figures in high relief, attached to a stone background; figures, seated or erect, attached to a block; figures supported by a dorsal column; figures in one solid piece, with the arms and legs symmetrical and united to the body, but not connected with any support; figures with the arms unsymmetrical and separate from the body, but the legs united and solid; and, finally, figures in dramatic attitudes, whose arms and legs alike are unsymmetrical and separate. In its fully-developed form, Sculpture consists of single figures or groups, in bronze or marble, having the natural colour of the material only, and representing for the most part the nude or semi-nude human form. This is the particular form of the art with which we must specially deal at present.

Though Sculpture is historically antecedent to Painting, yet it will be seen at once that it is more convenient to postpone its consideration to that of its younger sister-art, because it depends on many of the same sensuous, emotional, and intellectual gratifications, yet refuses the aid of others with apparent capriciousness. Nevertheless, this very refusal to call them all to its aid we shall find to be an important component in the special charm which Sculpture affords us.

Taking the same order of examination as before, we see that among the Actual Sensuous Pleasures Sculpture appeals to that of form alone. Colour it rigorously excludes. The reason for this rejection is probably as follows. The optical consciousness cannot readily be divided. Either it attends to form or it attends to hue; rarely and imperfectly to both together. If we take any simple æsthetic object, such as a vase, we shall see that when it is covered with coloured figures or flowers our attention is distracted from the general outline to the particular coloured shapes enclosed by it. If, on the other hand, its colouring is uniform, we think only of the beauty of form, leaving all other considerations on one side. Now, the perception of beauty-of-form we saw to be a higher æsthetic feeling than that of colour. Hence this deliberate sacrifice of the lower to the higher pleasure yields to those capable of appreciating it a gratification of unusual *purity*; thus importing into the estimate a vague emotional feeling. One of the most marked symptoms of the late æsthetic regeneration in England is the revulsion from gaudy Parisian taste in over-coloured and often ungainly vases to those of plain earthenware in exquisite shapes, either of a single uniform retiring hue, or of many varying shades in green and yellow, forming no definite pattern, but scattered iridescently over the surface; or, at most, having belts of black or darker ornamentation, marking what may be called the critical zones of the vessel, and so aiding the appreciation of its form. Similarly with animal shapes:

those which strike us most in respect to form are noticeable for the uniformity of their colour. Compare the Arab and the zebra, the puma and the jaguar, the gazelle and the fallow deer, the swan and the peacock. We see in each case that, even though the beauty of form is in itself nearly equal, the species which attracts notice by its colour thereby distracts our attention from its shape. So, too, ferns, the leaves whose form gives us the greatest pleasure, have no brilliant flowers to withdraw our notice from their delicate contour and symmetrical arrangement. Now, modern Sculpture depends for its purity upon just such a rigorous self-abnegation. The very word "statuesque," which we sometimes apply to living shapes, is an index of its true object. It aims primarily at affording us the highest pleasure of mere form, unalloyed by any considerations of colour. To do so, it chooses mostly that form with whose minute turns we are most conversant, the human body, and renders it in uniform marble or bronze. Accordingly, we derive more pleasure from nude statues than from draped ones, because then the graceful natural outline of the limbs is not masked by the clothing. Just in proportion as the drapery becomes stiff and cramping does the æsthetic value of the work decrease, until at last we get those hideous deformities in frock coats and trousers that inundate the public places of our manufacturing towns, in honour of successful cotton-spinners, to the utter demoralization of national taste and ethics. But the artistic superiority of the nude to the draped form gives an extra reason for the rejection of colour. Tinted statues, whatever may bè said about Hellenic precedent, offend the average modern taste, because they threaten the obtrusion of non-æsthetic sentiments. The coldness, hardness, and whiteness of marble limbs save them from any suggestion of the lower feelings; which, on the contrary, are inextricably bound up with the pleasures of colour and of soft warm touch. Occasionally animal forms may be represented in Sculpture: horses, fawns, lions, and panthers lend themselves well as subjects for the chisel, and the poised wings of a butterfly have been used with effect. Even elephants, camels, bulls, and dogs have been sometimes attempted. But we have not studied the minute morphology of animals with the same critical eye which we have turned upon the human shape; and hence the animals in Sculpture are usually mere accessories to the beauty of man or woman.*

The Ideal Sensuous Pleasure of suggested feelings is on the whole strikingly wanting in Sculpture. The thermal effect of marble is rather chilly than cool. Softness is conspicuous by its absence.† A female nude statue stands beautiful, but repellent. Occasionally, indeed, veils or drapery may suggest soft touch, but cultivated spectators feel that such tricks of art are inconsistent with that lofty self-abnegation which we have recognized as a principal charm of statuary. To beauty of form alone it elects to owe

* It may be objected that the view taken of colour in Sculpture in the above paragraph is contradicted by Dresden statuettes, and other porcelain figures. To this it must be answered that the pleasure derived from such productions is essentially different from that aroused by Sculpture proper. It is also one much lower in the æsthetic scale.

† Indeed, the hard texture of marble is one of its chief beauties. Sculpture imitated in plaster-of-Paris impresses us with the unpleasant idea that if scraped it will readily fall into a gritty powder.

everything, and to beauty of form it sacrifices every other mode of pleasure.

Ideal Emotional Pleasure is also of small importance in plastic art. The best pieces consist of single figures in repose. Composition distracts our attention from the form to the subject. It is true that a few emotional elements enter sparingly into certain great master-pieces; the sublime into colossal figures, the religious sentiment into sacred personages and winged angels, love (as a foregone certainty) into some compositions, pity into representations of wounded men or dying maidens. But in all these cases form is still the main element. It is the gracefulness of folded wings which suggests the angels. Without accepting in their entirety the views of Winckelmann, we may agree that marble is not a good vehicle for the expression of the emotions, because they depend so largely upon the eye, which cannot be properly represented without the aid of colour and chiaroscuro. So, that, on the whole, in spite of many great exceptions, those pieces of Sculpture please us most which give us the ideal nude form, in graceful attitudes, with distinction of permanent character in the cast of features, but without any attempt at the expression of mere passing emotions.

The Intellectual Pleasure of skilful imitation is present in Sculpture as in Painting. Yet even here there is a characteristic distinction. Though Painting, as a rule, selects only what is most beautiful in nature and rejects what is ugly, yet it may occasionally, for some effect of contrast or some special emotion, give us a deformed beggar or a litter of rotting vegetation. Sculpture, on the contrary, aims at absolute ideal beauty of form. Every limb must be in perfect proportion, every feature in exquisite harmony. As it mostly rejects composition, it cannot easily be led to introduce unpleasant figures for the sake of combinational effect. Moreover, any deformity, any mere ungracefulness, militates against that pure beauty of form to which Sculpture totally devotes itself. No skill can make the portrait-statue of a stout middle-aged gentleman in a surtout anything but shapeless and ridiculous.

Lastly, the Intellectual Pleasure of Plot-Interest is generally wanting to Sculpture. As it mostly rejects composition, it can tell only a very plain and simple story. There are a few pieces, however, like the Laocoon, which involve a certain amount of this feeling; and terra-cotta groups, which hover upon the border-land of Sculpture proper, often bear a close analogy to genre painting.

To sum up, Sculpture mostly differs from Painting in the very high and restricted order of pleasures to which it appeals. Its fastidiousness recommends it to the most delicate taste, and its austerity, its absolute remoteness from the warmer sensuous or emotional feelings, repels the less refined. Hence it usually lays itself out to suit only the most cultured classes, and rarely condescends to mere tricks of art or catchy emotional effects. Veiled ladies and crying boys always collect a throng at exhibitions; but artists linger before busts of Roman severity and female figures of more than Greek perfection.

Before we pass on from presentative to representative art,

from Painting and Sculpture to Poetry, there is one question which may naturally have occurred to the reader, and which it may be well to notice here. I have referred throughout to the beauty of the human face as a known fact, without any attempt to analyze it into its component factors. For this I have had two reasons. In the first place, it is very delicate ground to tread, involving complicated questions of sexual selection;* and in the second place, I think the subject has been productive of much error in earlier treatises. It is a common characteristic of awakening enquiry that it usually begins by attacking the most complex instead of the most simple phenomena. Thus, in physics, before men had settled the most elementary laws of motion, heat, or light, they constructed empirically the vastest a priori theories of the universe; in biology, before they knew the simplest physiological facts, they prescribed confidently for complicated diseases; and in mental science, before they had learnt anything as to the action of the five senses, they dogmatized on νοῦς and διάνοια, on conscience and free-will. Similarly in Æsthetics, long before anyone had endeavoured to account for the pleasurableness of red or blue, dialecticians exhausted argument on the nature of human beauty, with the general satisfactory result of proving that the features of Socrates were ideally lovely, or that sufficient early training would teach us to prefer the figure of a baboon to that of the Apollo or the Aphrodite. Now the fact is that human beauty is the most involved case in the whole range of

* See the whole difficulty fully set forth from this point of view in Chap. XIX. of Mr. Darwin's *Descent of Man*.

Æsthetic Feeling. Not only does it contain the most complex elements of form, colour, and symmetry, but it is further complicated by many emotional, intellectual, and ethical considerations. Moreover, it is largely affected by differences of race, class, family, age, sex, and individual peculiarities. It is, indeed, the instance where the largest allowances must be made for personal equation. Again, the fact that infants will answer sympathetically to the emotional expressions of pleasure or anger in others, prior to all experience of their meaning, shows that not merely the human face in itself, but even its passing modes, have produced hereditary connexions of nerve which answer immediately to pleasurable or painful stimuli. And further, we have observed and compared so enormous a number of human features and limbs that we can appreciate unconsciously all sorts of delicate varieties in contour which in any other subject would evade even the closest scrutiny. So minute are the points of discrimination that a passing indisposition, the shade of a bow, or the twist of one lock of hair, may make all the difference between prettiness and plainness. All that can be said with confidence is this :—human beauty is, in part at least, a combination of abstract pleasure in form and colour, with a certain given, relatively-rigid, symmetrical, normal, healthy type. All very wide divergence from the type is shocking to us, and is usually connected with disease, imperfection, or morbid function. But so long as the typical lineaments and distribution of colours are fairly well followed, we are pleased by such deft combinations of tints, such graceful curves and slender yet rounded limbs and features as would delight us in any inanimate object. Persons who for the first time mix with the African race in large numbers imagine, to begin with, that all are equally ugly, because there is so considerable a divergence from the European type: but as soon as the new standard has become familiar, those individuals who best conform to its ideal form, and who exhibit a lustrous deep-black skin, brilliant white teeth, clear and intelligent eyes, smooth, round, and glossy cheeks, flat but not very open noses, full and fleshy lips, with general plumpness of body, are recognized as handsome or pretty.* The men, however, though usually strong and muscular, strike a European eye as effeminate in their faces, owing to the smoothness of their skins, and the scantiness or absence of beard and whiskers. In the case of North American Indians, on the contrary, I notice that most Europeans consider the men handsome, noble-looking, and well-made, but that they regard the squaws as masculine and hard-featured. Here the type is so little removed from our own in many external points that we are able to appreciate its good characteristics at once: but the divergences are in some features so marked, and are of a sort so exactly opposite to those which give softness and sweetness to female faces in our own race, that we immediately associate them with the unlovely emotional elements of savage character. So that we must make great allowances for mere conformity to type in our estimate of human beauty; remembering that

* European artists who have not lived among the African race sometimes try their hands at a pretty negress ; but they always Aryanize the type, and so produce a face which looks, to one accustomed to living specimens, a mere ·ckly sentimentality.

appreciativeness for such conformity *may be* actually engrained in the nervous systems of each race. Of course, as already hinted, many other elements go to make up the total effect; and, on the whole, it seems best to leave the case of human beauty untouched, except so far as these few remarks may throw light upon it. It has only been alluded to here at all, because it is so prominent an element in the art of Sculpture that to pass it by without an apology would seem like ignoring a difficulty instead of candidly confessing that its complexity enables it practically to defy analysis.†

† A dissertation upon this subject will be found in Mr. Herbert Spencer's Essay on *Personal Beauty.* Mr. Spencer, however, mainly confines himself to ideal and emotional elements in the total effect, while I, in accordance with my general plan, have given greatest prominence to the immediate sensuous effect. At the same time I am most willing to allow that sexual selection and the survival of the fittest will in all probability have produced such an internal consensus that those persons of either sex who bear outward signs of intellectual, moral, and physical qualities adapted to their circumstances, and who are consequently the most desirable parents for the coming generations, will mutually please the opposite sex.

CHAPTER XI.

POETRY.

§ 1. *Æsthetic Nature of Poetry.*

Literature may be roughly divided into two great classes: that which aims at imparting knowledge, and that which aims at imparting pleasure:—in other words, the scientific and the æsthetic. In the first class may be included works on the natural sciences, on philosophy, and on history properly so called: to the second class we may assign Poetry, romance, and the mass of belles-lettres generally. Of course many kinds of writing hover on the borderland between the two: still, we usually recognize the fact that a book or a paper aims on the whole at one or the other of these two main objects,—the increase of useful information or the immediate gratification of the æsthetic sentiment. The purpose of science is of course equally to enlarge the happiness of men; but it does so by indirect means, and the pleasures which result from its cultivation can hardly be considered as æsthetic. With the first of these divisions we have consequently nothing to do; but the second falls naturally into its place in our present enquiry. It will be sufficient, however, if we examine the nature of Poetry, taken as a type of the class; since the pleasure felt in other imaginative literature has the same origin, and Poetry, being more exclusively æsthetic in its purpose than any other form of composition, embraces all the special points of other forms, besides a few almost peculiar to itself.

Literature has its beginnings far back in the infancy of man. History traces its origin to the sacerdotal annals of early Rome, to the knotted chronicles of Peru, and to the traditional pedigrees of real or mythical ancestors, up to Zeus and Woden, which form the boast of savage chiefs. Poetry dates back to the degraded myths which settle into fairy-tales and folk-lore, to the semi-religious epic of warrior life, and to the song of triumph which accompanies the dance of victory. In their beginnings, both are alike oral, and both alike differ very little from ordinary speech. Yet they are necessarily marked by some kind of assistance to the memory, which gives them their literary character. The proverbs, nursery songs, charms, and religious invocations of savage or semi-civilized peoples are either rudely metrical, or else contain rhyming lines and alliterative jingles. But as literature begins slowly to assume more formal shapes, a differentiation is gradually set up. That species of composition which vaguely foreshadows scientific writing is couched in the straightforward language of everyday life; that species which is simply æsthetic in its purpose, and which tends towards the production of modern Poetry, grows more and more confined to certain rules of material repetition, rhythmical recurrence, assonance, or alliteration. We have no difficulty in recognizing the song of Deborah or the ballad of Brunanburh from the midst of the chronicles in which they are imbedded. Side by side with the growth of this presentative pleasure, an ideal element is introduced in the stilted language, the ornamental tropes, the fanciful episodes, the emotional appeals to the joys of battle or the delights of the feast. Long before written Poetry begins, this double differentiation is carried out to a considerable degree of perfection. In the Homeric ballads, in the old English song of Beowulf, in the great Finnish epic, we get already regular systems of versification, a developed poetical phraseology, and the unmistakable æsthetic spirit. But it will be best for our present purpose, as with Painting, so with Poetry, to examine its structure in the most advanced form, which will necessarily include all the simpler modes of pleasure given by the earliest poems.

§ 2. *Presentative Elements of Poetry.*

The most conspicuous difference between Poetry and the other fine arts is this, that while they appeal directly to the eye or the ear, and aim only in a minor degree at emotional or intellectual pleasure, Poetry appeals very little to the senses, and owes most of its effectiveness to its ideal factors. But before we examine these proper poetical gratifications, we must glance very briefly at its presentative elements. It will only be necessary to allude to them in the most cursory manner, because they have been already mentioned under the head of Hearing. Poetry is generally distinguished from prose composition by some kind of rhythmical recurrence, either material as in Hebrew; quantitative, as in Latin and

Greek; accentual, as in English and German; or syllabic, as in French. It is also often marked by other modes of expected repetition, such as perfect rhyme, or assonance of vowels and consonants, found in most modern verse; imperfect rhyme, or assonance of vowels alone, which is the ordinary rule of Spanish poets; and alliteration, which is systematic in so-called Anglo-Saxon and Icelandic songs, while it is employed as an occasional beauty in all languages and ages. Besides these various mechanical devices, Poetry may further gratify the ear by smoothness of flow, which is obtained through high vocalization and the rejection of harsh consonantal combinations, awkward hiatus, and excessive sibilants or trills. Certain words are in themselves, apart from the suggested idea, harsh and disagreeable, while others are soft and pleasing; though of course these distinctions can only be observed by a cultivated and highly discriminative ear. Poetry seeks, so far as possible, to avoid the former and cumulate the latter: but this principle may be interfered with by considerations of intellectual or emotional effect. The various presentative elements thus shortly enumerated are commonly summed up as the *form* of Poetry, while the far more important representative elements, to which we next proceed, are known in contradistinction as its *matter*.

§ 3. *Representative Elements of Poetry.*

We all know that verse is not necessarily Poetry, and even that Poetry is not necessarily in verse. In reading fourth-rate rhymes we feel that they differ from prose only in their metrical arrangement. On the other hand, in reading certain impassioned passages of prose authors, we are often struck by a special emotional thrill, which we describe as poetical. What may be the nature and origin of this peculiar feeling is the question which we have to attack in the present chapter.

The medium through which Poetry gratifies the æsthetic sentiment is language: and in the great difference between language on the one hand, and colour, shape, and musical sound on the other, we have the groundwork for the distinction between Poetry and the sister arts. For colours, shapes and musical sounds, the elements of presentative art, are in themselves pleasurable stimulants to the senses: but words in themselves are seldom either pleasant or painful. Exception being made for the slight presentative differences mentioned above, their emotional quality depends entirely upon the object to which they are applied. They are symbols which, when heard or read, call up into consciousness a faint form of certain previously experienced sensations or emotions, singly or in groups. Thus the word *orange* calls up a vague and imperfect consciousness of the various sense-impressions which when actually present are known by that name. But words derive their power of gratifying the æsthetic sentiment from the fact that accompanying the faint form of the sensations which they arouse is a faint form of the appropriate associated emotion. Thus the word *lily of the valley* excites in us not only an ideal consciousness of the flower so called, but also a very slight wave of that pleasurable feeling which an actual lily produces in us through the senses of sight and smell. So, too, the words *violet* and *cabbage*, *palfrey* and *donkey*, *ruby* and *chalk*, do not differ very widely as to the manner in which they affect the auditory or optic nerves: but they are æsthetically gratifying or the opposite in virtue of the pleasant or unpleasant sensations, the dignified or undignified emotions, memories of which are aroused in connexion with the objects they symbolize. And if it be granted, as we saw to be probable, that the physical seat of ideal feelings is the same as that of the corresponding actuality, it will follow that the faint emotional waves generated by language exercise in a minor degree the same nervous plexuses which would be exercised more fully by the original vivid waves of which they are copies. We thus see how the pleasures of imagination can be finally affiliated on our general principle of pleasure and pain.

The ideal pleasures thus characterized may be aroused by single words in comparative isolation. Even in choosing names for persons or places we endeavour to select a title which shall convey some small amount of the emotional thrill. Thus we give our children the names of flowers, Lily, Violet, Daisy, Marguerite; or those of great mythical or historic heroes, Arthur, Alfred, Harold, Hector, Hugh; or such as call up some vague recollection of the imaginative past, Edith, Cyril, Eleanor, Ethel, Claude; or those belonging to characters in some favourite poem or romance, Rosalind, Beatrice, Cordelia, Dolores, Geraldine. So, too, with houses or estates: however questionable may be the taste displayed, there is at least an æsthetic intention in such titles as Myrtle Bank, the Cedars, High Cliff, Monloisir, the Nook, Nightingale Grove, and the thousand other sentimentalities of suburban villas. Now in all impassioned writing, such ideal sensuous or emotional feelings are occasionally and incidentally aroused in larger masses. But Poetry deliberately seeks to gratify the æsthetic sentiment by a conscious stringing together of ideas which give rise to the feeling of beauty. It lifts us into a fanciful atmosphere of sensuous and emotional delight, a land of perfect happiness, an imaginative realm where nothing common, base, or hateful is ever seen. Its object may be described as the attempt to arouse in the hearer the largest possible amount of massive pleasurable ideal æsthetic feeling.

We may consider the pleasures of Poetry under the same four heads which we examined in the case of Painting. But of these we have already dismissed the few presentative sensuous factors; and it will be convenient to divide the representative sensuous factors into two classes. So that our classification will be as follows: first, Simple or Abstract Ideal Sensuous Elements; second, Complex or Concrete Ideal Sensuous Elements; third, Ideal Emotional Elements; and fourth, Intellectual Elements. Each of these will demand a separate section.

§ 4. *Simple or Abstract Ideal Sensuous Elements.*

We have already seen in the earlier portions of this volume what special sensations are in the actuality gratifying. We have now merely to run through a brief list of them, in order to show that they can enter effectively into poetical composition just in proportion to their original pleasurable nature, and to their remoteness from life-serving function.

Beginning with the various senses in the order of æsthetic precedence, we come first to Sight. We saw that this sense has two principal functions, the perception of colour (including lustre) and shape. And we can now see that all beautiful colours and shapes are in the highest degree poetical. The names of all vivid hues are frequent in Poetry, such hues being themselves pleasant stimulants to the eye. As examples we may take *scarlet*, *crimson*, *pink*, *orange*, *golden*, *green*, *blue*, *azure*, *purple*, and *violet*. On the other hand, the names of dull and undecided colours are not in themselves poetical, the corresponding actualities not being remarkable for imparting any agreeable stimulus. Such names are *grey*, *brown*, *dun*, *black*, *bay*, and *drab*. It is true these words, like many others originally neutral, may become poetical by some effect of harmony or intellectual fitness: but these effects belong to the later consideration of the emotional and intellectual elements, and so cannot be examined here. One only has to read over the two lists to see how greatly they differ in poetical value. Again we saw that the red end of the spectrum, being less fully represented in nature than the blue, has acquired a greater pleasurableness as a stimulant: and we find accordingly that red and orange with their congeners are more adapted to Poetry (*cæteris paribus*) than blue and green with their cognate tints. That this is true will, I think, be clear to anyone who carefully compares the emotional waves roused by each of the words *crimson* and *azure*, or thinks of the number of passages in Latin Poetry where *roseus* and *cæruleus* respectively occur. The red sun, red gold, the red right hand of Jove, the red king Pyrrhus, ruby lips, cherry cheeks, ruddy faces, the rosy-fingered dawn, the crimson flush of eve, the scarlet stream of life, are poetical common-places. But it is a difficulty in making an estimate of the simple or abstract elements that the words denoting them are never used except as adjectives of a concrete, and that consequently intellectual appropriateness and skill of rendering have at least as much to do with the question as the original quality of the sensation. When we get to the concrete elements we shall see that this difficulty no longer besets us; that bright-coloured objects are more poetical than faint-coloured, and those in which red or orange preponderates than those in which green or blue takes the lead.

Passing on to the other mode of pure optical sensibility, lustre, we find that words denoting its presence are poetical, while those denoting its absence are not. Such are *brilliant*, *sparkling*, *sheeny*, *polished*, *lustrous*, *luminous*, *twinkling*, *glancing*, *silvery*, *pearly*, by the side of *dull*, *dingy*, *rough*, and *turbid*.

In the muscular element, shape, we saw that the motor apparatus of the eye is fatigued by sharpness, angularity, or intricate figures, while it is agreeably exercised by curved lines and harmoniously arranged forms. Hence whatever is *rounded*, *curling*, *graceful*, *lithe* or *flowing*, is more poetical than what is *straight*, *stiff*, *awkward* or *upright*.

So much for Sight. In Hearing, the next of the senses in æsthetic order, it will be observed that words denoting musical tones or harmonious combinations are poetical. Such are *clear*, *ringing*, *silvery*, *musical*, *sweet*, *melodious*, *mellow*, *rich*, and *low*. Those of an opposite nature are (unless redeemed by some other effect) unpoetical. Such are *shrill*, *hoarse*, *grating*, *harsh*, *loud*, and *croaking*. It may, however, be mentioned that words denoting varieties of sounds are frequently transferred from other senses, and so carry with them much of the associated feeling which is gained in their original sphere.

In Touch, the emotional element is weak, the perceptional taking the lead. Hence words relating to this sense are neither very poetical nor the reverse. But its few emotional aspects are ideally reproduced in Poetry, affording us the adjectives *soft*, *waxen*, *fleecy*, *smooth*, *delicate*, and *tender*, in contrast with *hard*, *rough*, *harsh*, *tough*, and *coarse*.

In Smell, which is an exceedingly emotional sense, the distinction is very marked. *Fragrant*, *sweet*, *perfumed*, *scented*, *odorous*, and all other words denoting pleasant sensations of smell are highly poetical: while those denoting ill odours, such as *stench*, *stinking*, &c., are so intensely unpoetical that they almost defy introduction into Poetry unless strongly recommended by intellectual effects or emotional association. For example, a poet might in a strong passage say of some practice (for instance, slavery) that it "stank in his nostrils;" but the expression is only endurable, first, because it harmonizes with the violent tone of disapprobation, and secondly because it has been sanctioned by familiar use in the English Bible, and has thus acquired a complex emotional effect.

In taste may be adduced such words as *sweet, sugared, luscious, melting, delicious, honeyed,* in contrast with *bitter, sour, biting, acid, rough,* and *acrid.* It is to be noticed that this sense, which is in the actuality eminently unfitted for æsthetic purposes on account of its connexion with necessary vital processes, becomes poetically possible in the ideal, but only in those of its forms which are least intimately allied with the digestive process, and which we classed as Tastes Proper; while those species which, after Professor Bain, we called Relishes and Disgusts, being closely connected with digestion, are inadmissible in any shape.

Lastly, amongst the organic sensations, all such words as *cool, fresh, buoyant, warm, easy, pure,* and those relating to health, repose or sleep are poetical. *Hot, close, weary, cold, chilly,* and words relating to disease, hunger, thirst, or restlessness are the opposite, unless redeemed by special connexion with some complex emotion.

It must be carefully noted that in all these cases nothing more is asserted than that the words are (or are not) in themselves elements of Poetry, apart from peculiarities of context. But in the division to which we next proceed, the compound or concrete sensuous elements, this difficulty will no longer be felt, and it will be seen that every concrete object is capable of entering effectively into Poetry just in proportion as it combines a large or a small number of the above-mentioned pleasurable sensations.

§ 5. *Complex or Concrete Ideal Sensuous Elements.*

Amongst concrete objects which enter into the composition of Poetry, visual qualities are the most important. The rainbow and the tints of sunset owe their poetical efficiency to colour alone. With the addition of lustre, we have the diamond, pearl, ruby, sapphire, beryl, emerald, amethyst, and gems in general: to all of which we shall have hereafter to add an emotional element of costliness. Dewdrops, jet, amber, coral, and ivory may be placed in the same category. If with these we combine beauty of form, we get the flitting butterfly, the gorgeous humming-bird, the crested peacock, and the waving plumage of the bird of Paradise. The beauty of man and woman, though intermixed with a large emotional element, is partly referable to the same source; hence we may include here rosy lips, vermeil-tinted cheeks, golden locks, snowy brows, and waxen arms. And by the further addition of perfume, we get all the wealth of summer flowers; the blushing rose, the dainty violet, the orange blossom, the nestling lily, the proud carnation, and the luscious clover in the scented meads.

To form almost alone are due the poetical efficiency of architecture and sculpture. Here are to be placed the palace, the temple, and the cathedral; the arch, the column, and the architrave; the swelling dome, the airy pinnacle, the star-ypointing pyramid, and the tapering spire: though in all these, again, large allowances must be made for the emotion of the sublime and the religious sentiment. Under the same head also we may include those plants and animals into whose beauty colour does not largely enter; such are the hind, the doe, the greyhound, the leopard, the eagle, and the swan; the elm, the ash, the palm, the ivy, the linden, and the vine.

Sound makes up for sight in the lark, the linnet, the throstle, and the nightingale. It also supplies the poetical element to the harp, the lute, the lyre, the flute, the trumpet, and the clarion; to music generally, Cecilia's varied world of sound, liquid treble and thundering bass; the distant bells, the lowing kine, the hum of the bee, the murmur of that eternal zephyr, and the rippling of the water in the flags.

Touch contributes to the concrete elements of Poetry chiefly in combination with other senses. Soft and yielding objects, such as wax, down, the marble forehead and glistening shoulders of Glycera, a baby's arm, owe part of their poetical effectiveness to their tactual properties. Smoothness, too, adds beauty to gems, polished stone and crystal, as well as to certain leaves and the human skin. On the whole, however, this sense, not being a specially emotional one, does not enter largely into the ideal factors of Poetry.

Taste gives us honey, wine, and milk, besides innumerable fruits. We may select as good examples (embracing other senses as well) the grape, the apple, the plum, the citron, the pomegranate, and the olive. Golden jellies, lucent syrups, sparkling juleps, combine beauty of colour with delicacy of flavour. But this, the most monopolist and functional of the senses, is subject to the special limitation which was noticed and explained above. The boldest of poets could scarcely venture to introduce roast goose or apple dumpling.

To the class of organic sensations we may refer cool grottos (which are a legacy to us from the south of Europe) summer breezes, evening with its stillness and fresh zephyrs, groves and mossy couches, sleep and drowsiness, rest after labour, and the whole poetical furniture of the *Lotus Eaters* and the *Castle of Indolence.*

In all these cases we can easily refer the poetical effect to some one or two separate senses; but there are other concretes in which all the pleasurable feelings seem inextricably united so as to defy complete analysis. As these contain the greatest possible numbers of agreeable sights, sounds, smells, tastes, and other sensations, besides combined emotional factors, they are of course the most poetical of all; that is to say they rouse the largest volumes of ideal pleasure. Such are the vast assemblages of objects which make up a beautiful landscape or impressive pageant. Mountain glens, hemmed in with beetling rocks, through which white foaming streams rave ceaselessly; woods and valleys, pastures and meadows dappled with daisies, sweet with the breath of kine, vocal with the song of birds; an Italian lake, bathed in sunset glory, its overhanging terraces rich with autumn tints, while a rainbow spans the tiny cataract that plashes musically into its unruffled bosom, and the soft sound of the vesper bell steals over it from some neighbouring campanile, half hidden amid chestnut and orange-blossom; far above whose green heads the roar of the thunder and the flash of the lightning play awfully around the pinnacles of eternal ice—these are a few of the great concrete wholes with which Poetry deals, whose elements can be sifted and referred to their proper place as we read them over, but which would scarcely repay the toil of a minute and deliberate classification.

Before proceeding to our next division, the emotional elements, it will be well to consider what results we can derive from our analysis of the sensuous factors alone. The reader will observe that on attentively conning over any of the above lists, or still better some familiar descriptive passage in his favourite poet, he is conscious of a faint emotional wave, varying in intensity according to the number of pleasurable sensations ideally aroused. He will also notice that while each word does not *definitely* bring up into consciousness all the æsthetic points possessed by the object symbolised, it does so *indefinitely*. While the word *ravine*, for example, does not awaken a complete picture of the object so called, nor a full recollection of the accompanying gratification, it awakens a vague consciousness of the object, with a correspondingly vague emotional thrill. This thrill it is the office of the poet to arouse, to sustain, and to economise. It is because each thrill is separately not very strong that I have defined the purpose of Poetry as being the production of *massive* pleasurable emotion; using the word in Professor Bain's sense, as opposed to *acute*. Poetry depends for its effect upon the unbroken succession of beautiful ideas and images, not upon the separate result of individual impressions.

Again, it will naturally result that each class of sensations will enter efficiently into poetical composition just in proportion as it is capable of being easily and distinctly recalled into consciousness on the suggestion of the words which symbolise it; and capable also of arousing in a faint form the appropriate emotional feelings.*

Now of all our senses Sight is the one which best admits of being reproduced ideally in the form most nearly resembling its original vividness; and after Sight in this respect comes Hearing. Accordingly, the greater part of the sensuous elements of Poetry consist of ideal visual sensations. Poetry is mainly pictorial, and much of its art is, to use the well-chosen modern phrase, word-painting. If we wish to convey the notion of a given scene to the mind, we can do so most fully in terms of Sight, and the mind is capable of realising the scene to itself in such terms far more readily than in any others. Sounds are also readily recalled, and consequently rank next in poetical value. Odours, while less retainable, have moderate persistence, and their strong emotional character makes them valuable adjuncts to the poet. But touches yield so little pleasure or pain, and taste and the lower senses are so little revivable, that they hardly occupy any appreciable place in the colour-box of the versifier. Moreover, they are often open to a special objection which must next be considered.

As the object of Poetry is to arouse the largest possible volumes of the ideal æsthetic thrill, it will follow that any set of sensations or any object which is pleasurable only in one aspect, while it is painful in another, will be unfit to

* Hence that preference of the concrete to the abstract, and the particular to the general, which has long been recognised as one of the empirical rules of poetical composition.

enter into verse composition. This is often expressed as a general rule of artistic technique by saying that the pleasure must be *pure* or *unmixed.* If a plant or animal be beautiful to the eye but possess a disagreeable odour, it will not be a fit subject for Poetry, because the unpleasant idea of smell will be suggested at the same time with its pleasant form and colour. The insufferable skunk is as graceful and glossy as a marten. So again an object which is delicious to the taste may be ugly to the eye, or a bird of lovely plumage may possess a discordant note. In these cases, if the object be introduced at all, care must be taken to suggest only its pleasant aspect, to the exclusion of its disagreeable side and where this cannot be effected, its name must be given up as hopeless, and removed without appeal from the poetical vocabulary. There are many emotional difficulties complicating this question, such as the effect of antiquity, novelty, or poetical prescription; for the present it will be sufficient to approach it from the sensational side alone. Now the act of eating and many others of the lower processes have æsthetically disagreeable adjuncts which unfit them for introduction into Poetry, unless redeemed by an appeal to other senses, and by directing the attention rather to the beautiful appearance of the objects than to their actual taste. If the gustatory sense be introduced at all it must be in the form of allusions to delicate flavours and dainty discriminations of bouquet, not to the coarser and more animal pleasures of food. The Homeric satisfaction at abundance of roast meat and drink jars upon modern ears. We all feel that dessert is the Poetry of dinner—not, indeed an

English dessert of raisins and almonds, sweet biscuits, and dry figs, but a painter's southern table, laden with pine and melon, peaches and pomegranates, oranges and grapes, laid out on massive silver, and set off with red wine dancing in the slender flagons. (In Poetry wine is of course usually red.) An example or two may serve to illustrate this principle. Milton says of Adam's table,

> "Eve within, due at her hour, prepared
> For dinner savoury fruits, of taste to please
> True appetite, and not disrelish thirst
> Of nectarous draughts between, from milky stream,
> Berry or grape."

And again,

> "So saying, with dispatchful looks in haste
> She turns, on hospitable thoughts intent
> What choice to choose for delicacy best,
> What order so contrived as not to mix
> Tastes not well joined inelegant, but bring
> Taste after taste upheld with kindliest change.
> . . . . . Fruit of all kinds, in coat
> Rough or smooth rind, or bearded husk or shell,
> She gathers, tribute large, and on the board
> Heaps with unsparing hand; for drink the grape
> She crushes, inoffensive must and meaths
> From many a berry; and from sweet kernels pressed
> She tempers dulcet creams; nor these to hold
> Wants her fit vessels pure; then strews the ground
> With rose and odours from the shrub unfumed."

Keats, too, thus describes the supper in the *Eve of St. Agnes*:

> "He from forth the closet brought a heap
> Of candied apple, quince and plum and gourd,
> With jellies, smoother than the creamy curd,
> And lucent syrups tinct with cinnamon;
> Manna and dates in argosy transferred
> From Fez; and spicéd dainties every one
> From silken Samarcand to cedared Lebanon."

And, once more, here is Tennyson's picnic at *Audley Court:*

> "There, on a slope of orchard, Francis laid
> A damask napkin wrought with horse and hound;
> Brought out a dusky loaf that smelt of home,
> And, half cut down, a pasty costly-made,
> Where quail and pigeon, lark and leveret, lay
> Like fossils of the rock, with golden yolks
> Imbedded and injellied."

Now in all these passages (omitting for the present the emotional elements of costliness, antique allusion, oriental tinge, or primitive innocence) the poetical feeling is entirely due to their picturesque character. The objects are not described as food but as parts of a scene. In itself a game pie is vulgar and inartistic enough, appealing to a sense which is both monopolist and closely connected with vital function; but the skill of the artist is shown in overcoming the difficulty by presenting the pie to us in such a light that we see only its beautiful pictorial points.

So too, with sexual feeling. Closely bound up as it is with our most powerful complex emotions, it yet defies introduction into Poetry, because the feelings aroused, though they may be pleasurable, obviously fall short of æsthetic disinterestedness. It can only be introduced under a veil of mysterious reverence, as in the well-known love passages of *Paradise Lost.* Even on those only a Milton could have ventured.

It may be added before we proceed to the emotional division that descriptive poems, as well as the greater part of narrative verse, are chiefly composed of sensuous factors; though no high-class poem can be so entirely. The *Georgics* and Thomson's *Seasons* may stand as cases in point. Mere lists of beautiful objects often produce a genuine æsthetic thrill. What can be more poetical than the catalogue of precious stones in the foundations of the New Jerusalem?—the jasper, the sapphire, the chalcedony; the emerald, the sardonyx, the sardius; the chrysolite, the beryl, the topaz; the chrysoprasus, the jacinth, the amethyst. And yet it is only a catalogue after all. Milton is peculiarly happy in rapid strings of names for natural objects, and Shelley's *Alastor* consists of little else than separate gems of scenic description, strung on a slender thread of connecting narrative. But there is always more or less of human emotion as well, or else the verse sinks from Poetry into the mere oriental profusion of the *Arabian Nights*. On the other hand, however emotional the main theme, it must be dressed up in copious simile, metaphor, and other devices for introducing the sensuous elements, or the verse will appear poor, frigid, and colourless.

Lastly, it is worth notice that while sweet sounds, meadow scents, and other sensuous elements are originally chosen as factors of Poetry because of their intrinsic pleasurable nature, yet their ideal employment in verse re-acts upon the actuality, so that our pleasure in their positive perception is mixed up with literary and poetical recollections. A mis-interpretation of this fact led to the fanciful theories of Alison and Jeffrey.

§ 6. *Ideal Emotional Elements.*

The complex emotions, which form only occasional components in the pleasure derived from Painting and Sculpture, enter into the very essence of Poetry. For we saw in our chapter on the subject that ideal emotion approaches much more nearly to the actuality than ideal sensation. Accordingly, language can gratify us far more by calling up subjects of pleasurable emotion than by mere word-pictures of agreeable sights and sounds. Even those concrete objects which formed the theme of the last section are constantly raised into the sphere of higher imagination by some fanciful emotional touches bringing them into comparison with complex human feelings. Thus the rainbow and the sunrise reappear as Iris, the many-hued, and Aurora, the rosy-fingered. Personification, or the attribution of mental qualities (especially emotional) to inanimate objects, is one of the ordinary devices of Poetry. We speak habitually in verse of the modest daisy, the flaunting daffodil, the gladsome light of day, the eager cataract, and the angry murmur of the thunder-cloud. Sleep glides gently down from heaven upon our wearied eyelids; Famine stalks gaunt and hideous through the land; Confusion and Flight march in the conqueror's van, with Sorrow's faded form and Solitude behind. In all these instances allowance must be made for intellectual factors; but a considerable residuum of feeling is due to the special emotions. Thus, in a joyous piece we make all nature rejoice with us; in a meditative one we see calm reflexion in every object about us. We may properly enquire, therefore, in connexion with our present subject, what complex emotions are of a pleasurable sort, and what poetical elements they afford. In dealing with this question it will be best to depart from the strict order of psychological arrangement, and to place first those emotions which are most frequently employed in the composition of Poetry. And first we may consider the emotion of the Sublime.

The Sublime takes its origin in admiration for literal physical greatness, and, in its very earliest developments, the greatness of the strongest men. It is thus closely akin to the sympathetic pleasure of manual skill. The members of a tribe naturally make much of the strong man who guards them from the enemy, and the deft-handed man who fashions for them arrow-head and hatchet. Hence arises a delight in feats of strength, which is gradually transferred to the deeds of mythical ancestors; to imaginary beings, gods and djinns; and again to inanimate objects, mountains, rocks, the cataract, the ocean, whose vast size and enormous force are contrasted with the puny thews and limbs of mortal men. Next, it is extended to remote time, the dim past, the greatness of duration; to remote space, the vast universe, the greatness of extension; to thought, genius, the greatness of intellect; at last to moral grandeur, heroism, the greatness of ethical endurance. We find, consequently, that the earliest Poetry, the ballad literature of savage tribes, is almost wholly engrossed with the mighty deeds of heroes in battle; when relieved at all, it is by the acts of the great gods and the majesty of natural scenery. The *Iliad* rests its much exaggerated claims upon these grounds. It will be seen that the passages which strike us most and cling longest in the memory are those which appeal strongly to these early germs of the Sublime:—the Titans piling Pelion upon Ossa; Phœbus Apollo, like to the night, coming down from the peaks of Olympus, wrathful in heart, the arrows clanking in the quiver on his angry shoulders; or Achilles, sitting apart, looking over the illimitable sea, wine-coloured, harvestless, while big scalding tears of rage and shame roll down his burning cheek. We get a great advance on such mere material conceptions in the Prometheus of Æschylus. Every line is gigantesque, yet sustained in its majesty by the sense of ethical self-sacrifice. On the snow-clad crags of Caucasus the strongest of the gods binds down the mightiest of the Titans in chains of adamant, to suffer tortures ineffable, infinite, godlike, undeserved: yet even in that inexpressible agony the unconquered soul stands glorious in its consciousness of right, fulminating curses unabashed against the reckless despot of the universe.

But, to come down to detail, we must see how these various developments of the Sublime help to compose the elements of Poetry. All such adjectives as *great*, *vast*, *huge*, *mighty*, *awful*, *boundless*, *infinite*, *eternal*, or *sublime* are in themselves highly poetical. Huge limbs, stalwart frames, gigantic might, are the *point de départ*. In superhuman creations of the imagination we have Zeus and Briareus, Thor and Odin, Sin and Death, with the whole mythological machinery of epic generally. Amongst animals we may adduce the lion, the tiger, the pard, and the war-horse,* aided of course by sensuous elements of form and colour: as well as the huge earth-shaking beast, and that Leviathan which God of all his works created hugest, neither of whom have such original advantages. All natural scenery

* See the Book of Job.

depends largely on the Sublime for its impressiveness: whether in the sombre pine or giant oak, the mountain and the crag, the river and the ocean, the Alps and the Himalayas, Ætna breathing fire or Niagara clad in spray. Architecture, too, besides beauty of form, owes a great share of its effect to massiveness and height: so that we may include here part of the feeling produced by the mention of lofty domes and towering minsters, the rock-hewn temples of India and the endless colonnades of Nile. Moral heroism fills as yet but a small area of the poetical field, yet its employment is probably becoming more frequent. Borrowed grandeur gives us the more vulgar elements of royalty and rank; king, queen and emperor; knights and dames; palaces, courts, and castles; jousts and tournaments; rich brocade and cloth of gold. Chivalry is especially poetical, for, in addition to greatness of rank and ascribed moral qualities, it is set off by time and poetic prescription. High-born maidens, the pomp of power, the lordly castles where the wealthy nobles dwell, are all referable to this head. The last example leads us on to costliness, which is of immense use to the poet, appealing strongly to a form of admiration which all can understand. Jewels, beautiful in themselves, become all the more poetical on this account. The adjectives *golden*, *silvery*, and *pearly*, implying attributes themselves sensuously efficient, are employed far oftener than their intrinsic value would justify, owing to the superadded emotional wave generated by the idea of wealth they remotely suggest. It is easy to recollect cases where *golden* is applied to fields of corn, wines, human hair, lightning, sunset, and autumn leaves; not omitting golden hopes, golden youth, or the golden prime of good Haroun al Raschid. Clouds lit up by sunlight are spoken of as molten gold. Silvery is similarly used of the moon, the hair of the aged, the shimmer of the sea, the sound of bells, or the laughter of lovely women. Try to substitute *yellow*, *grey*, or any other appropriate epithet in these cases, and see how instantly the æsthetic effect is diminished or disappears entirely. So, too, we have ruby lips, the sapphire sea, the emerald isle, and the pearl of women, besides jetty locks and ivory brows. Compare also the frequent use in Poetry of the words gem, crown, and diadem in metaphorical senses, and of king or prince to denote mere preeminence.* Antiquity, the Sublime in time, adds also to æsthetic effect. All that is venerable, ancient, time-honoured, commands our admiration. The antique life of mediæval Europe, baron and knight and paladin, steward and seneschal, page and vassal, hall and bower, are antiquated in language as well as in fact. Mr. Tennyson has made good use of the mysterious halo through which the Arthurian legend looms larger than human. Solemn cloisters and mouldering colleges, though less ancient, are quite old enough to strike

* The reader must remember that I do not suppose the notion of costliness to be definitely present to the mind either of the poet or his audience; but merely that an indefinite emotional wave due to that cause has become associated with the word, and is brought up into consciousness along with it. The poet, dimly aware of this wave, seizes the word as being best adapted to his purpose, and judges it, as his critics judge it, not by itself, but by the general effect which it produces along with many others in a sentence. The business of the analyst is to reverse this process, and trace back to its ultimate components that massive and highly compound thrill which the whole verse arouses in our minds.

the mind with their grandeur on the score of age alone, even without the myriad associations which gather round their ivy-clad arches and dust-encrusted gargoyles. On the other hand, new objects, machinery, the steam-engine; modern drinks and perfumes; scientific phraseology; words of recent coinage, are, from their very newness, unpoetical. American Poetry is seldom of modern America. Longfellow revels in the old Rhineland and the peaceful Flemish towns, or if he finds a native theme, he goes back to the Puritans of Plymouth, the habitants of Acadia, or the ancient Indian legend of Hiawatha. New York and Boston are too new to versify. I instanced above, under smell, myrrh, nard, and frankincense; but we could hardly add, Jockey-club, millefleurs, or frangipanni. By the side of the lute, the lyre, and the guitar, the fiddle and the piano find no place. Modern chemical nomenclature is too precise, definite, and unimaginative; the poet's medicine chest contains only the primitive remedies, oil and wine, balm and honey. As a drink, too, wine, the most ancient of stimulants, is highly poetical; but we cannot say as much for rum and beer.*

* It would encumber the text too much to enter fully into the respective values of wine and rum, but the following analysis may perhaps be permitted in a foot-note. Wine is the juice of the grape, an exquisitely-coloured purple fruit, whose delicate foliage and twining tendrils have every beauty of form and symmetry. It grows on the sunny hills of Rhineland, or the green volcanic slopes of Campania, and its vintage is connected with dark-eyed Provençal maidens—with village holiday or sacred festival of Dionysus. Its poetical hue is ruby-red or amber-coloured, and the sunlight dances merrily through its beaker. Its perfume is almost as soft as flowers. It is found in every book of the Bible, on every page of Greek or Roman verse. It is itself, in classical song, a very god; the poet is inspired by the bodily indwelling of

Here there are numerous other elements, sensuous and emotional, which complicate the question; but we get the naked effect of time in the contrast between honey and sugar. Hence it is that Poetry clings to archaic forms and obsolete modes of spelling. The second person singular is more poetical than the plural; preterites such as *spake*, *drave*, and *clomb* are preferred to their modern equivalents; and even *rime*, *ladye*, and similar archaisms are considered by a certain class of poets as prettinesses.* Especially poetical are words which have been consecrated by employment in early ballads, and more particularly, to Englishmen, those which are frequently found in the authorised version of the Bible. Other considerations, however, of the domestic and religious emotions come in to eke out this feeling; and, on the other hand, novelty often gains more praise than antiquity. It is impossible, indeed, to make divisions of the elements which will not in part overlap one

Bacchus; and even for the austere Hebrew muse, it maketh glad the heart of man. It is sanctified by the holiest rite of the Christian Church. It has, in fact, every claim of actual or ideal sensuous pleasure, of sacred or profane emotional association. Rum, on the contrary, is the produce of the rigid sugar-cane. It is grown in new lands and unhealthy climates, by the aid of slave labour or degraded negro cultivators. Its colour is dingy and turbid; its scent is strong and disagreeable. In flavour, it lacks refinement; the fiery spirituous element is strong and rough, the gentler delicacy of bouquet is altogether wanting. It is a modern commercial product; it is associated with sugar-broking and distilleries; it has no sacred or poetical prescription, but is connected in thought with vulgar boisterous drunkenness and London public-houses or police-courts. It has every disadvantage, sensuous and emotional, besides being designated by a curt and uneuphonious monosyllable. Consequently, while the former word brings up by its mere mention a whole flood of pleasant ideas, the latter is utterly inadmissible into Poetry because of its cumulative disagreeable adjuncts.

* See also Mr. Herbert Spencer's Essay on *Use and Beauty*.

another; for, inasmuch as the object of the poet is to call up the greatest possible volumes of the æsthetic thrill, he employs by preference those expressions which appeal to the greatest possible number of senses and emotions: and it is consequently difficult not to bring up the same instances time after time under different heads. The complete analysis of the thrill which accompanies the word "cathedral," for example, could hardly be accomplished under several pages.

There is a special case of the emotion of the Sublime which it is worth while to mention before passing on. I mean the employment of numbers to give an idea of vastness, power, or duration. A hundred, a thousand, a million, have each their poetical value. Myriads are both numerical and vague; centuries definite but imposing. Seventy times seven is biblical, and contains the sacred number which has not even yet lost its charm. Three and thrice are small but mystical.

Second in this class ought to come the emotion of the Ridiculous, which is a pleasurable one, and might therefore be supposed at least allowable as an element. Yet we find it rigorously excluded. The reason is to be sought in the principle of harmony. The Ridiculous is utterly opposed to and destructive of the Sublime, which always enters largely into Poetry. It has been well defined by Professor Bain as the sudden degradation of a person or thing possessing dignity. Hence verse which is sustained for a certain length of time and intentionally collapses is rightly considered, not as Poetry, but as a distinct species of composition, comic verse. An unintentional and unconscious collapse of the same sort is *bathos*, the worst of all technical blunders. The ridiculous jars upon us and puts us out of tune for the beautiful. Don Juan sins terribly in this respect. Its finest passages are constantly disfigured by the intrusion of disgusting images. It is owing to a similar reason that whatever is low, mean, or impure must be banished irrevocably from Poetry, as from all fine art.*

The next class to be considered is a somewhat heterogeneous one, which in an ultimate analysis would have to be very much subdivided and redistributed, but which for our present purpose may be considered as one and single. We may call it the sympathetic class, using the word in a much wider sense than usual, and comprehending under it three principal heads; the emotion of Pity, the Domestic Feelings, and the Amatory Passion.

The first division, Pity, is an agreeable feeling of an opposite origin from the Sublime. As that consisted in the admiration for what surpasses ourselves, this consists in the pleasure of protecting what is weaker and smaller than ourselves. All that needs aid, support, assistance; all that is shrinking, clinging, helpless; finally, by analogy and transference, all that is small, dainty, delicate, calls forth the sentiment. Originating in the parental and marital relation, it spends itself primarily upon human objects, women, children, babes at the breast, the aged and infirm; next, it extends itself to dumb animals, the faithful dog, the harm-

* Upon this subject the reader may be referred to Mr. Herbert Spencer's Essay on the *Physiology of Laughter*.

less, necessary cat, Lesbia's sparrow and Burns' mouse especially to tiny species, such as humming-birds and lap-dogs: lastly, it is transferred to works of art, wee flowers, the shrinking violet, the clinging eglantine, and the lily nestling in the glade. Words expressing minuteness are consequently poetical. Diminutives are very useful to Latin and German versifiers. Catullus revels in them: his little ode "Ad Coloniam" is worth reading in this connexion. The emperor Hadrian's "Animula vagula, blandula," is untranslatable. Verbs of endearment convey a notion of weakness and relative smallness: such are *cherish*, *dote*, *fondle*, *nestle*, and *cling*. The ivy, pity-struck, clothes the dying oak, and the vine weaves its tendrils round the sturdy elm to which it is classically wedded.

The last division merges insensibly into the Domestic Emotions, from which it takes its origin. The names of all the closer family relationships are in themselves a mine of poetical wealth. Father, mother, brother, sister, each call up a deep and stirring thrill, which is rendered all the purer æsthetically by its disinterested character. Home and hearth, the old familiar faces, the sacred name of friend, are also powerful in their degree. The Domestic Emotion is the chief inspiring muse in Macaulay's picture of an old Roman fireside (in *Horatius*), where the chestnuts hiss in the embers and the kid turns on the spit: and it enters on a larger scale into *Hermann und Dorothea*, *Evangeline*, and *Dora*. Here, too, we may place the objects which long association has made part of our lives. The little English wild-flowers, not very brilliantly coloured and often destitute of perfume, the daisy, cowslip, primrose, buttercup, sweet briar, and violet, are yet of wonderful emotional potency; for we have gathered them from childhood upward in the green hedgerows at home. Perhaps the reader was disposed to enquire, as we glanced at the brilliantly-coloured tropical birds, why toucans and macaws could not compete with such familiar little friends as linnets, robins, thrushes, and sparrows: but (omitting their powers of song) that the latter are little gives us half the solution, and that they are familiar the other. This feeling must be added to that of the Sublime, mentioned before, as making the language which has been long used in Poetry or enshrined in the English Bible peculiarly impressive. Gorgeous descriptions of southern scenery, like the island in "Enoch Arden," or the shining Orient of "Locksley Hall," may dazzle us with the brilliancy of their colouring and the richness of their luxuriant ornamentation; but they do not speak direct to the heart like Wordsworth's daisy or Shelley's skylark. The elements of the one are almost purely sensuous, of the other almost purely emotional. Of course Poetry may be written about places and objects with which we are not familiar; but to make it effective it must have some compensating emotional element, or at least sensuous points of unusual vividness and variety.

Here perhaps should be interpolated the feeling of Patriotism, which is the extension to the tribe or the nation of sentiments originally roused in the narrower limits of the family. *Patria, Fatherland; Zion, Hellas, Italy;* all have their appropriate thrill. Even the word *English* is often highly poetical, as in Marvell's "English boat," and Tennyson's "Sweet English lily." We can throw ourselves sympathetically into the position of other nations and read with a borrowed patriotic glow the sonorous trimeters of the Persæ, the magnificent outburst of Italian nationality in the second Georgic, or the stirring songs of Körner.

The Amatory Emotion has much in common with the Domestic Feelings. It is hardly necessary to add that it is the most poetical in our whole nature, for it is the most complex and the most all-embracing: and it is a feeling of peculiar strength and vividness. Examples need not be given at length, as two-thirds of all Poetry bears witness to its power. In classical authors, however, the sensual side of the passion is most dwelt upon; in modern, the emotional. As extremes, we might take the *Ars Amatoria* and *Maud.* The so-called Anacreon is utterly devoid of feeling, a mere voluptuary; and even Catullus, though his passion is genuine, all-absorbing, and wonderfully earnest for his age and race,* yet belongs distinctly to the heathen world. That loveliest of love poems, Acme and Septimius, is the full outburst of hot untrammelled youth in an age that was not ashamed of mere sensual display. The modern rejection of such elements is paralleled by the abandonment of colour in sculpture; and the late effort in France and England to revive the earlier treatment is decidedly an æsthetic retrogression, like Gibson's attempts at tinted statuary.

The Religious Emotion has much in common with the Sub-

* But perhaps he had a touch of Keltic blood.

lime, and is also partly cognate to the Domestic Feelings. Leaving out of consideration its direct employment in devotional Poetry (which can hardly be treated of here, where we are engaged with æsthetics alone) it enters largely as an indirect component into ordinary verse. All words connected with worship, such as *church*, *prayer*, *psalm*, *hymn*, *orison*, and *litany*, convey a faint echo of their sacred sense. *Cathedral*, *temple*, *chapel*, *minster*, *altar*, *nave*, and *dome* have already appeared in other connexions. Sabbath bells are beautiful to the stanchest Protestant, while vesper chimes carry us away to mediæval cloisters or Italian hill sides. The pealing organ and the vaulted aisle both give and take solemnity from their religious use. Even more decidedly religious references may produce a good effect if they harmonise with the subject and are not unnecessarily obtruded. Once more, the language of the Bible must be mentioned under this head.

The Ethical Sentiments are not as yet sufficiently differentiated from the Religious Emotion to require separate treatment. Yet we may perhaps specially notice the peculiarly pure thrill which we receive from what we call "a noble thought" in verse.

The purely Egoistic Feelings enter but little into the composition of Poetry, except in alliance with more sympathetic affections. They obviously lack the required disinterestedness. Self-complacency is only a subject for Poetry when treated dramatically, as in *St. Simeon Stylites* and the *Northern Farmer;* in which case the pleasure derived from it must be handed over to the Intellectual class. The Irascible Affection is allowable when kept within certain limits and directed to a proper end, or what the poet and his audience consider as such. In conjunction with Patriotism or political feeling it becomes a powerful adjunct. Macaulay's pictures of Appius Claudius and Sextus Tarquinius are blackened with hatred and contempt which almost rise to sublimity; and when we read of the latter that "wriggling in the dust he died, like a worm beneath the wheel," we lower ourselves for a moment to the level of the fifth century in our glow of cruel satisfaction. Appeals to such feelings were common in the old martial and anti-social Poetry, but are dying out as sympathies widen. The fierce Homeric χάρμη is giving way to psalms of love and brotherhood.

Finally, we have to examine one very strange and abnormal phenomenon of Poetry, as of all other arts, the occasional employment of painful sympathetic feelings as an æsthetic stimulant, which is the essence of what we call *Pathos*. The question thus raised is a very difficult one, and cannot be adequately answered except in an extended essay. A few considerations, however, may be briefly mentioned here. In the first place, unselfishness is an idea closely bound up with our highest conceptions of æsthetic pleasure; and from unselfishness to pity, from pity to Pathos, the step is very slight. Again, pathetic scenes, pictorial or literary, strike us more with intellectual admiration for the skill of the artist than with direct emotional pleasure: when pushed too far, the feeling becomes positively painful. But, above all, we feel that Pathos is requisite in art, because otherwise it would strike us as too childish and unreal. Depth, earnestness, tenderness, all our higher feelings, must be gratified by art, unless it wishes to sink to the level of Eastern tales or children's stories.* During the present century the desire for this melancholy tone in art has steadily increased, and the reason why is clear. Man stands to-day, as he never stood before, face to face with the naked realities of nature. Solitary in a boundless universe, alone on a little isthmus of historic time between the vast sea of vague geological æons and the unknown future of cosmic cycles, he finds himself awe-struck and ignorant, ready to fall prostrate before the terrible forces of nature, which work out unswerved their fatal will in apparent disregard of his happiness or misery, of his prayers or imprecations. No wonder that, in such circumstances, we can feel but small interest in mere pictures of daily enjoyments. No wonder that we cry like infants for the light and fling our weight of cares upon the great world's altar stairs that slope through darkness up to God. *In Memoriam* only echoes the cry of the century.

§ 7. *Intellectual Elements.*

The various factors of Poetry which have been hitherto enumerated bear much the same relation to the completed poem as the canvas and colour-box of the painter bear to his completed picture. They are only the parts out of which the final total is built up. The pleasure derived from the composition as a whole, though largely emotional, is also to a great extent intellectual. A mere unorganised collection of these various elements would not be Poetry but its raw

* See an admirable Essay by Mr. Sully in *Mind* for October, 1876.

material. The earliest poems are scarcely more than unconnected episodes, gathering loosely round the myths of Achilles, Beowulf, or Krishn Chand: there is no composition, no poetical perspective. But as art advances a closer connexion is required between the various parts. Thus, at last, every poem becomes an organic whole, with due subordination of parts, and a single consistent thread of argument, whether it be of a circumstantial tale, as in epic, dramatic, and narrative verse; or a pictorial scene, as in descriptive verse; or a thought or conceit, as in lyrical and epigrammatic verse. The poem is the expression in language and amplification in detail of this primitive conception. In following such a work we have wide opportunities for the gratification of the Intellect.

First amongst the class of Intellectual pleasures in Poetry we may place Plot-Interest. This is the sustaining thread of epic and narrative poems, and enters largely into the drama. It acts in Poetry precisely as it does in Romance. When too exclusively relied upon, however, it tends to obscure the æsthetic elements, and to obliterate the distinction between Poetry and Romance proper. The great literary revolution begun by Goethe and Schiller, Scott and Byron, consisted largely in the increased importance attributed to Plot-Interest. It is generally absent from the most purely æsthetic form of verse, the lyrical.

Next may be placed the pleasure of skilful imitation. This feeling is closely analogous to our admiration for careful execution in pictorial art. A good description of an object in itself indifferent is commended by its fidelity; just as

Wilkie's blind fiddlers and village dames, though not in themselves beautiful or interesting personages, yet charm us by their naturalness and reality. Poetry, like Painting, has improved immensely in truthfulness since its earliest days. The first poets deal only in a few stock æsthetic objects, to which they merely allude without special description. Roses are their only flowers, the lark their only bird: red gold, ladies gay, the green wood, the gallant steed, reappear in every ballad. There is a conventional epithet for every noun; the white-armed, the cloud-compelling, the laughter-loving, the grey-eyed; and these are always employed, however incongruous the context. The colours are almost as primitive and as unshaded as those of the Egyptian paintings. Homer knows only three or four; the Attic poets enlarge the stock; Latin verse gets to some dozen; while the modern poet subdivides by all the known tints, by all the precious metals and stones, by all the flowers and leaves, by sky and sea and human features. So, too, with natural scenery: the early poets give us only a few broad touches; Wordsworth works up with minute care every vein in a leaf, every petal in a flower. Who has not admired the intense faithfulness of those lines of his?—

> "Would that to this small daisy's self were known
> The beauty of its starlike shadow, thrown
> On the smooth surface of this naked stone!"

Or Tennyson's description of a village maiden's hair,

> "In gloss and hue the chestnut, when the shell
> Divides threefold to show the fruit within."

Indeed, unpopular as the opinion may be, I do not hesitate to say that Poetry, as an imitative art, has advanced as far above the Homeric level as Painting has above the Egyptian. And I do not base this statement upon mere individual taste, but upon a careful comparison of epithets, descriptions, similes, and metaphors. The composers of the early Hellenic cycle were doubtless wonderful versifiers for their age; but they belonged to *their* age, not to *ours*.

Here should be referred the principal pleasure of Dramatic Poetry, which consists in watching the life-like and accurate development of imaginary characters. Indeed the Drama may almost with greater propriety be regarded as a department of Romance than of Poetry in the strictest sense.

Next to this gratification derived from a consciousness of truthful delineation and vivid colouring may be placed the pleasure afforded by ingenuity on the author's part. Such purely Intellectual interest carries us through the Ovidian prettinesses and the frigid couplets of the English Augustan age. It even casts a false glitter over the laboured reams of Erasmus Darwin. Sometimes it rises higher and affords us a more genuinely æsthetic thrill, as in the clever collection of instances from antiquity which surprise us on every page of *The Princess*:—Vashti and Sheba, Joan of Arc and Artemisia, Cornelia and Sappho, the Oppian Law and the pleading of Hortensia. Virgil and Milton pride themselves on being learned poets. Here, too, may be placed the use of scientific and metaphysical conceptions, which has been gaining ground of late years. United with the feeling of the Sublime, and appealing to interests daily increasing in diffusion, they will doubtless form in the future a powerful æsthetic instrument.

Before concluding it should be added, to guard against misconception, that although it has been necessary for purposes of analysis to begin with the simplest factors, the synthetic process of composition follows exactly the opposite order. The main idea must come first; the verse must be its embodiment. The poet does not begin by taking up a handful of elements, and then combine them into a poem: he strikes out his poem first, and then dresses it out with the elements. But in working out this original rough sketch the elements above enumerated (or some amongst them) must be employed and harmoniously combined. If they be neglected, however good may be the original design, the result is mere prose; the æsthetic thrill is not adequately sustained throughout. Furthermore, the conception as a whole must itself appeal to one or other of the pleasurable emotions. The dominant feeling may be pity, love, domestic affection, patriotism: but unless there is some one thread running through the whole, we get a rambling, disconnected stream of "spasmodic" images, instead of a consistent poem. Thus the whole as a whole, and each part as a part, must yield æsthetic gratification. Poems rich in decoration but wanting in depth or continuity disappoint us; as Scott said of Mrs. Hemans, they have too much foliage and too little solid wood. On the other hand, poems such as Samson Agonistes, fine in their original conception but without sufficient ornamentation, are heavy and bald. They stand like bare oaks in winter, imposing but not beautiful. Moreover, each incident must be not only in itself æsthetic, sublime, or emotional, but must also contribute to the general effect, or at least not conflict with it. Poetical skill is shown in nothing more than in preparing the mind of the reader and bringing it into harmony from the beginning with the dominant emotion of the piece. The first few stanzas should strike the key-note; the remainder should keep up the sentiment once aroused. A splendid example of this may be seen in the introduction to Poe's *Raven*. Every possible circumstance of mystery and weird melancholy is brought to bear upon us before the actual supernatural actor is introduced upon the scene. Choice of time and place are important in the same regard. Most short reflective poems open with a few descriptive stanzas which serve to bring the mind into unison with the tone of the whole. In this branch of his art the poet derives much assistance from the various devices of metre and rhyme.

Before concluding this chapter let me meet one objection which is certain to be raised against this analysis. Where, it will be asked, in such a system, is there room for Genius? If Poetry consists merely of such special combinations of such special elements, why cannot any man sit down and write a great poem? The answer is that poetical genius *is* the power of thus combining and arranging these elements. Not every man has his mind so stored with the beautiful and sublime objects of external nature, with the noble and pathetic emotions of the human heart. Not every man can so adorn whatever subject he touches with grand images and eloquent words. Let us take a parallel from a sister art. Painting is merely the combining of certain colours and shapes in accordance with certain laws. Any man may learn them and recognise their truth. But only the born artist has the power to employ them in the production of great pictures. Only the born artist has the imagination to group together his ideal figures, the eye to catch the faint harmonies of light and shade, the hand to trace those delicate tints and graceful curves which make up the glorified countenance of a Madonna. So it is with the poet. First in his mind rises vaguely the conception of some touching tale or some stirring lyric. Next comes the spontaneous choice of a metre that harmonises with his theme. Gradually he shapes his idea and fleshes it out with episode or sentiment. Finally he selects for every stanza and every line the loveliest and choicest words or pictures, drawn from the inexhaustible stores of his memory and his imagination, where he has gathered together, as in a treasure-house, all that is glorious and beautiful, without and within, in the boundless universe or in the soul of man. The total result so obtained is that harmonious and noble work of art, a Poem.

THE END.

BRADBURY, AGNEW, & CO., PRINTERS, WHITEFRIARS.

Made in the USA
Monee, IL
04 November 2026

67385003R00164